Break Through
Your
Set Point

Break Through Your Set Point

How to Finally Lose the Weight

You Want and Keep It Off

George L. Blackburn, M.D., Ph.D.

with Julie Corliss

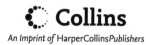

Collins

An Imprint of HarperCollinsPublishers

To my wife Sue, with eternal love and gratitude

HarperCollins books may be purchased for educational, business, or sales promotional use. For information please write: Special Markets Department, HarperCollins Publishers, 10 East 53rd Street, New York, NY 10022.

Illustrations on pages 8, 15, 85, 104, and 105 were done by Scott Leighton. Graphs and drawings on pages 23, 45, 95, and 182 were done by Susan Morreale. The Healthy Eating Pyramid on page 107 was done by Christopher Bing.

FIRST EDITION

Designed by Level C

Library of Congress Cataloging-in-Publication Data

Blackburn, George L., 1936–

Break through your set point: how to finally lose the weight you want and keep it off / by George L. Blackburn with Julie Corliss. — 1st ed.
p. cm.
Includes bibliographical references and index.
ISBN 978-0-06-128867-8
1. Weight loss. 2. Physical fitness. 3. Nutrition—Popular works. I. Corliss, Julie. II. Title.

RM222.2.B5828 2007
613.7—dc22   2007026056

08 09 10 11 10 9 8 7 6 5 4 3 2 1

Contents

Acknowledgments

This book, which my patients and colleagues have asked me to write for years, embodies the knowledge and experience of not only my own research but that of many experts in the areas of weight loss, nutrition, and exercise. In addition to those mentioned in the book, I would like to pay tribute to my mentors, Paul Schloerb, William McDermott, George Clowes, JP Flatt, and Vernon Young, whose work helped to establish the field of nutritional medicine. All of my colleagues, fellows, and students know that this is a truly multidisciplinary effort. I would especially like to extend my thanks to Bruce Bistrian and to all of the Harvard faculty and visiting faculty, who tirelessly help with the Harvard Continuing Medical Education course on the practical approach to the treatment of obesity.

The collaboration with my coauthor, Julie Corliss, arose from a ten-year-long stint working together on *HealthNews*, a consumer publication from the Massachusetts Medical Society. Julie's experience as a seasoned medical writer was an essential ingredient to this book.

Two trusted and highly proficient research assistants, Belinda Waltman and Katie Wang (both of whom went on to medical school), provided much-needed support both in organizing information and providing insightful edits on the many iterations of each chapter. Many thanks go as well to Barbara Ainsley, our operations manager, whose skill, dedication, and patience keeps our division running smoothly, and to Rita Buckley, our medical editor. We also owe a debt of gratitude to our clinical research dietitian, Kristina Day, who provided key information and guidance for Chapters 5, 6, and 9, and to exercise physiologist and assistant professor of medicine at Harvard Medical School, Dan Rooks, who reviewed and improved Chapter 7. Charles Davis, a physical therapist, also shared his experience and expertise in Chapter 7. Miriam Simun's thoughtful comments helped us clarify our message in the book's early chapters.

I wish also to thank Mickey Stunkard, a lifelong friend and colleague, whose silhouettes provide invaluable guidance and reference throughout the book, and Tom Wadden, who carries on his work at the Center for Weight and Eating Disorders at the University of Pennsylvania. Further gratitude is sent to the following colleagues, who graciously agreed to review chapters within their areas of expertise, including Louis Arrone, Steve Berrien, David Blackburn, Kelly Brownell, Gary Foster, Isaac Greenberg, Ned Hallowell, Steve Heymsfield, Ed Horton, Jim Hill, Chick Koop, Ethan Sims, and Walt Willett. I would also like to acknowledge Herb Benson, David Heber, Lee Kaplan, Robert Kushner, James Levine, Chris Mantzoros, Barbara Rolls, Allan Walker, Brian Wansink, and Rena Wing, whose efforts to promote nutrition, metabolism, and behavior proved instrumental in the development of this book.

Special thanks go to our agent, Doe Coover, who helped us to shape and sharpen our central message and provided steady encouragement throughout the book's creation. Kathy Huck, Ryu Spaeth, and Lelia Mander, our editors at HarperCollins, also deserve many thanks for their thoughtful comments and edits, which invaluably strengthened this book.

Finally, I would also like to acknowledge Danny Abraham, my best friend and founder of the Slim Fast Food Company, whose generous support helped to establish both the Center for Healthy Living within the Division of Nutrition at Harvard Medical School and my endowed chair in nutrition medicine at Harvard. Danny's enthusiasm and healthy lifestyle (his eating and exercise habits are exemplary!) also provided inspiration during the three-year-long creation of this book. With his words, I lead you to the start of this book.

One of the most exciting days of my life was in November of 1976. That was the day when my brother-in-law Dr. Ed Steinberg and I visited with Dr. George Blackburn at his Boston apartment at approximately eleven o'clock at night. That was the only time he had free to see us, and we were not going to pass up on the opportunity to meet the world's greatest nutritionist!

We were just embarking on the launching of SlimFast, which was in those days just a fortified protein powder. SlimFast was used in place of meals, so it needed to be nutritionally balanced and complete. Meeting with George was not only exciting, but also rewarding—and very educational for us.

Slim Fast became what could only be described as the world's most complete and balanced food, thanks to George's original and continuous education. Just about everything we know about good nutrition, weight loss, and good health was due to our relationship with George. He is an inspiration. I hope that you enjoy reading and benefiting from this book as much as Ed Steinberg and I enjoy living the life that George inspired us to live. Eddie is 88, and I am 83. With George's guidance and healthy living advice, we both expect to keep going for a long time to come.

Introduction

You know the feeling: cranky, tired, and hungry—the telltale signs of another diet attempt gone awry. Whether you're dealing with a recent middle-age spread or a lifetime of being too heavy, chances are you're desperate to lose weight to look and feel better. But despite your best efforts, you aren't succeeding. Perhaps you've hit a plateau and can't seem to nudge down the number on the scale. Or maybe you've managed to reach your goal weight only to regain the pounds.

Failing at weight loss isn't due to a lack of awareness, money, or effort. We know that being overweight can lead to health problems. Dieters join weight-loss groups, start and abandon diets out of frustration, and buy the miracle products pitched in magazines, on television, and on the Internet. Each year, Americans spend an estimated $50 billion on weight-loss products and services. Despite this enormous cash outlay, two out of every three people in the United States are overweight, and about half of those are seriously overweight or obese.

In our convenience-driven society, abundant food and fewer opportunities for physical activity make it easy to gain weight. Some of the blame also lies with the overhyped marketing of fad diets and dietary supplements that promise to melt fat away. Infomercials and Internet ads imply that you can lose weight with little effort. It's hard to abandon all hope of a quick fix when new products and new diet plans continue to promise amazing results. If you're reading this book, you may already know those claims aren't true. And with more than thirty years of clinical experience in helping patients lose weight, I can say with certainty that there's no such thing as a magic bullet.

I tell my patients that while it isn't easy, it *is* simple. You don't need to give up any of your favorite foods, and you don't have to count calories. To lose weight and keep it off, you need to follow three steps:

1. Eat less food.

2. Eat healthful foods.

3. Be physically active.

Here's the novel part: *Set a reasonable goal to lose about 10% of your initial body weight. Then hold steady at your new weight without regaining any weight for at least six months, which will reset your body's set point (or typical body weight).* Once you've reset your set point, you can repeat the cycle to lose even more weight. Following this advice in the context of a structured daily routine will reap positive changes in your health, well-being, and appearance and prevent those extra pounds from coming back. I'll show you how managing your time more effectively and getting more sleep can help you accomplish these goals.

I know you've heard the basic message many times before: eat less and exercise more. What's different about *Break Through Your Set Point* is that it gives you specific tools and targeted advice to effect and sustain those changes. The book you're holding includes all the tips and tricks I've prescribed to my own patients to help them restructure their eating and exercise habits and lose weight. Most importantly, I never give any weight-loss patient the exact same advice, because each person has unique reasons for gaining weight and making lifestyle or behavior changes. But whether you're a busy parent with kid-food syndrome (you eat chicken fingers and sugar-coated cereals on a regular basis) or you're a former athlete-turned-couch-potato (your exercise routine fell by the wayside after you left school), this book will help you devise a plan that works for you.

One of my mantras is find your own path and take the journey slowly. This easy-does-it approach isn't a concession to laziness. My program is based on the proven scientific fact that the body resists losing weight after a certain point, which stems from the body's innate tendency to protect itself against starvation.

This book is based on three decades of my own research and clinical practice, coupled with innovative findings from other experts in the field. My doctoral studies at Massachusetts Institute of Technology (MIT) identified the twenty-plus essential nutrients required in special formulas used to deliver nutrients through a vein. This type of feeding, known as total parenteral nutrition, nourishes and sustains people who are unable to eat normally because of gastrointestinal surgery or other problems. My expertise in this area prompted a request from a physician and a businessman to develop a formula for a good-tasting, nutritionally sound meal replacement that people could buy over the counter to help them lose weight. This became the SlimFast shake, which has proven to be a safe, effective weight-loss aid not just in clinical trials but also in a long-term study.

During my surgical training at Kansas University, I witnessed and studied the dire complications of early weight-loss surgeries. With the help of Dr. Edward Mason, who developed the Roux-en-Y gastric bypass procedure—a vast improvement over the previous surgeries—I introduced this technique to the Boston area in 1975. It is now the most commonly performed surgery for treating severe obesity.

The most meaningful discoveries I've made deal with the range and rate at which people lose weight and how those factors affect their regaining the weight. My studies were the first to discover that most people can change their body weight by only 15 to 20 pounds at a time. I demonstrated that this modest loss will improve health, helping people to recover from weight-related problems such as diabetes, high blood pressure, and high cholesterol. Countless other studies by researchers around the world using a variety of different diets confirmed the same phenomenon, which has formed the basis for national guidelines now promoted for the treatment of overweight and obesity.

We know that the body imposes a natural limit on how much weight you can lose. It is governed by an internal balancing mechanism that works to keep your body weight at a stable point—or set point. My studies documented that people failed at weight loss only when they tried to lose too much weight too quickly and without long-term goals. They also showed that diet was only one facet of enduring weight loss. It took a multidisciplinary team approach with dietitians, behavioral therapists, and health care providers to enable patients to eat less, choose healthy foods, become physically active, and achieve a lifelong healthy body weight.

As you are introduced to the set point theory, you'll learn how your genes affect your set point and explore the myriad of environmental influences that have caused Americans' set points to creep upward over the past few decades. You'll see how the 10% solution is governed by your set point, and more important, why this modest weight loss is enough for most people to become healthy and stay healthy for years. I will lead you through the lifestyle changes that will help you realize the three simple steps of eating less, eating healthy, and exercising more. The case studies will help you identify your own challenges around food, activity, time management, and sleep. By mastering a simple journaling technique that allows you to track your progress, you can figure out which areas to target and adopt strategies that resonate for you. In essence, this book provides the pragmatic program that will get you lasting results.

I've spent decades investigating the treatment of the diseases linked with both starvation and excess weight. I've helped thousands of patients. But there's another reason you can trust me, which is that I really do know how you feel. I used to be 20 pounds heavier. I was not blessed with a naturally fast metabolism. I make choices every day that help me stay at a healthy weight. Nearly every morning, I take a brisk 2- to 3-mile walk around the pond near my home. Afterward, I leisurely spend twenty minutes enjoying a healthy breakfast of cereal, fruit, and skim milk, eating slowly to give my stomach time to tell my brain that I'm full and satisfied. My office is on the eighth floor of the hospital, and I walk up those flights at least once a day, often twice. My lunch usually consists of a big salad with dark, leafy greens topped with vegetables, nuts, dried fruit, and raspberry vinaigrette. These choices are now second nature for me, like brushing my teeth. I stick with these patterns not just because they prevent me from gaining back that 20 pounds but also because I know they'll keep me healthy, fit, and feeling great.

Society as a whole—and doctors in particular—have become keenly aware of the need to prevent many diseases linked to excess weight. This book offers a holistic, lifelong prescription to address this need. Given today's environment, resetting the average American's inflated set point is a tall order. But by working with our families, workplaces, and communities, we can do better. I hope this book can help incite this transformation—one that I'm confident will lead to successful weight loss, better health, and happiness for all those who try it.

The Science of the Set Point

It is one of the great wonders of the brain that body weight stays remarkably fixed (as a "set-point") most of the time in most people.

—Christian Broberger, M.D., Ph.D.,
Department of Neuroscience,
Karolinska Institute, Stockholm, Sweden

The drive to regain is mainly in the brain.

—Barry E. Levin, M.D.,
professor of neuroscience,
New Jersey Medical School,
East Orange, New Jersey

WHAT IS A SET POINT?

Your body weight set point is the number on the scale your weight normally hovers around, give or take a few pounds. Your heredity and your environment—starting back at the moment of your conception—determine your set point. Most people's set point is "set" around age 18. Before that age, your body is still growing, and you need to eat more calories than you burn to encourage growth and development. Girls may reach their set point a little before age 18, and boys may reach theirs a bit later. But soon after you stop growing in height, your body weight tends to settle at a fairly stable number.

Your set point doesn't necessarily remain the same throughout your lifetime. Few of us weigh the same as we did when we finished high school, and that's perfectly normal. As you age, your metabolism slows down a bit, which is why most people put on a few pounds. Additionally, women normally gain about 25 to 35 pounds during pregnancy. If they don't lose most of that extra weight within about a year of giving birth, they're likely to raise their set point, especially if that trend continues during future pregnancies.

Gaining just under a pound or so per year from about age 20 to age 50 is common and not necessarily bad for your health. People get into trouble when they gain more pounds more quickly, ending up at an unhealthy body weight. Over the long term, excess food and insufficient exercise will override your body's natural tendency to stay at its set point and lead to a higher, less healthy set point.

What's My Silhouette?

In addition to a body-weight set point, everyone has a silhouette that closely parallels their body shape. A chart developed in the early 1980s depicts a range of body sizes, from slender to obese. Used as a research tool to examine people's perceptions of their own body image (both actual and desired), the silhouettes provide a close approximation of a person's body weight. In effect, your silhouette is a visual representation of your set point.

I will use eight of these images for each gender as a simple way to help you see how you can change your silhouette to a healthier profile by resetting your set point. Take a close look at these silhouettes and circle the one that most closely resembles your body now. What about your silhouette at age 18? (Note that these silhouettes were developed using Caucasians, so they may not accurately depict your body if you have a different racial background. But overall they provide a close approximation for most people).

Easy Come, Not-So-Easy Go?

Researchers who study weight control have discovered that people who gain weight easily find it hard to lose extra weight, but people who struggle to gain weight find it easy to lose excess weight. A slow, grad-

MALE

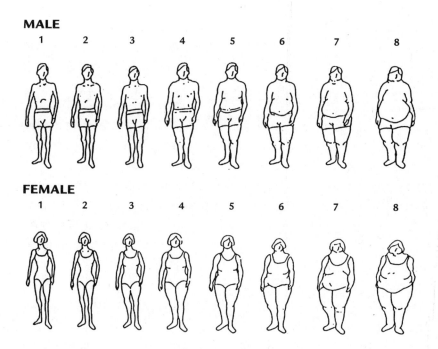

FEMALE

The average American moves from silhouette 2 to silhouette 4 between the ages of about 20 and 50.

Source: Reprinted with permission. Stunkard, AJ, Sorensen, T, and Schulsinger, F. Use of the Danish Adoption Register for the study of obesity and thinness. *Res Publ Assoc Res Nerv Ment Dis* 60 (1983): 115–20.

ual weight gain will fool your body into thinking that your set point should be higher—and, in fact, that *does* reset your set point. For instance, a 20-pound weight gain over several decades moves you from silhouette 2 to 4. Then when you try to lose weight, your body defends that higher weight, making weight loss more difficult. On the flip side, a rapid, short-term weight gain doesn't fool your body and therefore does *not* reset your set point. Your body will work to defend its lower, normal set point, and shedding those excess pounds will be relatively easy.

But just as it's possible to reset your set point to a higher point, it's also possible to lower it. The secret is to work with, not against, your body's natural tendencies and lose weight slowly, one silhouette at a time.

HOW YOUR BODY SETS YOUR SET POINT

To appreciate how your body works to maintain your weight, it helps to understand a little bit about the internal controls that govern this complex process. These controls include a tiny structure deep within the brain, nerves that run between the brain and the stomach, and a host of hormones. Central to this entire system is your metabolic rate, which automatically adjusts in an effort to maintain your set point. (But, as you'll learn later, external forces can override these internal controls.)

Making Sense of Metabolism

Metabolism refers to the basic chemical processes within the body that keep you alive. It's also vital to understanding weight control. During the periods of the day when you are not eating, proteins, carbohydrates, and fats are broken down into their building blocks, creating energy to fuel all your body's functions, while other processes consume these substances. Your metabolic rate is a measure of how fast your body uses that energy, or burns calories, when you're at rest, just lying quietly and not doing anything. Also known as your resting energy expenditure (REE), this number accounts for about 70% of the calories you burn each day. On average, this comes out to about 10 calories per pound of body weight.

REE varies from person to person and changes throughout life. It is mainly influenced by several things you can't control: your genes, your age, and your sex. Your energy metabolism slows down as you age, a natural consequence of the body's cells wearing out and not functioning quite as efficiently. Men tend to have a slightly higher metabolic rate than women, although a woman's will (not surprisingly) rise temporarily during pregnancy.

The Internal Speedometer

The remaining 25% to 30% of the calories you burn are from any physical activity you do, from simply fidgeting in a chair to taking a walk or doing vigorous exercise. It's the only aspect of your total energy metabolism (or total daily energy expenditure) you can control. Think of your metabolic rate as your own internal speedometer. Say you burn 1 calorie per minute lying down. Sit up, and you're now burning $1\frac{1}{2}$ calories per minute. Stand, and you're up to 2 calories per minute. The more you move, the more you burn. These seemingly trivial increases can make a difference over time. You need to burn more calories than you take in to lose weight. That's why it's so important to be active throughout the day. Just 100 of the 2,000 to 2,500 calories you consume each day can mean a difference of 10 pounds of body weight from one year to the next!

What about all those advertisements for dietary supplements that promise to boost your metabolism? Don't waste your time or money believing these false promises. There is absolutely no scientific evidence that any substance can significantly rev up your metabolism. The only safe and effective way to boost your metabolism is to burn more calories by picking up the pace and moving around more.

The Thyroid Connection

The thyroid, a butterfly-shaped gland that wraps around your windpipe, secretes hormones that regulate your metabolic rate. If you've gained weight recently, someone may have told you to have your thyroid level tested. It's true: low thyroid levels, a condition known as hypothyroidism, can cause symptoms such as fatigue and weight gain. But this problem, which can be diagnosed with a simple blood test, is rarely the underlying cause of weight gain.

The Hypothalamus: Headquarters of the Set Point

About the size of an almond, your hypothalamus sits atop your pituitary gland at the base of the brain, just above the roof of your mouth. This well-protected location speaks to the vital importance of this brain region. In addition to controlling hunger and satiety, the hypothalamus keeps the body in balance, a process known as homeostasis (from the Greek *homeo,* meaning "like" or "similar," and *stasis,* meaning "standing still"). This internal balancing mechanism regulates your body temperature, as well as the amount of sugar, salt, water, and other substances in your bloodstream.

Most of the time, your temperature stays right around normal, or 98.6 degrees Fahrenheit, because the hypothalamus sends and receives a series of chemical messages that regulate your body temperature. It's somewhat similar to the thermostat that controls your home's heating system: When the temperature drops, the thermostat sends a signal to turn on the furnace. Likewise, if you're cold, the hypothalamus checks in with other sensors in your body to see how it compares with the set point. If your temperature is lower than the set point, it sends a signal to your muscles, telling them to contract. That causes you to shiver, which helps you warm up. Conversely, if you're too hot, you sweat, which helps you cool down. The body reactions happen involuntarily, without you even having to think about them. They're perfect examples of your autonomic nervous system at work, which also plays a key role in homeostasis and your set point.

The Autonomic Nervous System

All the nerves in your body that extend beyond your brain and spine belong to the peripheral nervous system. The autonomic nervous system (ANS), which controls the organs and muscles inside the body, is part of that network. Most of the time, we aren't aware of the workings of the ANS, since it usually works in an involuntary, reflexive manner, widening or constricting your blood vessels, raising or lowering your heart rate, or prompting your intestines to move and digest your food.

The ANS is most important in two situations: It responds immediately in emergencies that cause stress, requiring us to "fight" or "take flight" (that is, run away). The ANS also works during nonemergencies, relaying messages that allow us to "rest and digest." Of course, this system is constantly acting to maintain the body's normal internal working, which is why it's an integral part of the set point.

Sending Signals: A Host of Hormones

A wealth of research has helped us understand more about the signals that talk to the hypothalamus to control body weight set points. They include the hormones insulin, leptin, adiponectin, ghrelin, and others.

The pancreas, an organ the size of a small banana that lies near the stomach, secretes insulin. Insulin controls the amount of glucose in your blood by moving it into the cells, where this fuel can be used by your body for energy. Leptin, which is produced mainly by fat cells, contributes to long-term fullness signals by gauging the body's overall energy stores. Yet another hormone, adiponectin, is also made by fat cells and involved in body-weight regulation, apparently by helping the body respond better to insulin and ramping up metabolism. Ghrelin, the so-called hunger hormone, tells the brain the stomach is empty, prompting hunger pangs and a drop in metabolism. Gastric bypass surgery (in which surgeons convert a person's stomach to the size of a small egg, effectively bypassing most of the stomach) doesn't just help people eat smaller amounts of food. The procedure also triggers a sharp drop in ghrelin levels, which lessens hunger and apparently contributes to the weight-reducing effects of gastric bypass. Traditional dieting, however, tends to boost ghrelin levels.

The Sensing Stomach

The stomach communicates with the brain through the ANS, and the nerve of interest to our story is the vagus nerve (see illustration). In Latin, *vagus* means "wandering," an accurate description of how this vitally important nerve travels from the brain to the stomach. When filled with food or liquid, the stomach's stretch receptors send a message via the vagus nerve to the brain that says, "I'm full!" Have you ever no-ticed that eating a large, heavy meal can cause you to perspire? That's the vagus nerve working overtime. As discussed, the autonomic ner-vous system prepares the body for fight or flight by raising your heart rate, increasing your blood pressure, and causing you to sweat. So by eating too much, you've made your body ready for fight or flight, even though you're just sitting at a table eating dinner!

THE VAGUS NERVE

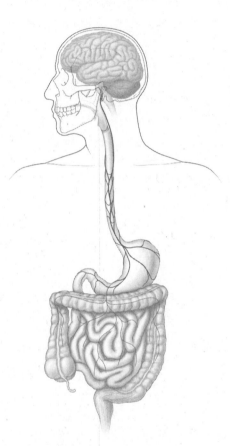

Originating in the brain stem, the vagus nerve extends down through the neck to the stomach and intestines.

Not surprisingly, most weight-loss aids (in addition to surgeries) focus on fooling the body's natural tendency to hold on to weight, mostly by manipulating levels of brain chemicals. Back in the 1950s and 1960s, dieters took amphetamines, which speed up metabolism by boosting the activity of the sympathetic nervous system. But they're also addictive and have many unpleasant side effects, including paranoia and heart problems. (For more information on weight-loss medications, see the Appendix).

Obesity as a Metabolic Disease

The reason weight-loss medications can't provide any real results is that we have a complex, overlapping system of checks and balances that help "defend" our body-weight set point. Many different genes contribute to your body weight, and thus it's impossible to manipulate it by focusing on just one hormone (or other substance). Others will jump in to compensate. The brief explanation of leptin and the other major players in this defensive strategy barely skims the surface of this intricate system. The take-home message is that these factors are beyond your conscious control. Our broader understanding of these factors has dramatically changed the framework of how we view the problem of weight gain and obesity. Instead of thinking of obesity as the consequence of a lack of restraint or willpower, it's now increasingly recognized as a disease that results from a breakdown in the body's normal system of checks and balances.

WATCHING THE SET POINT AT WORK

Now that we know how the set point works, let's step back and take a look at some of the other evidence in support of the set point theory. These observations include both short- and long-term studies and anecdotes from people in a variety of different settings.

The Framingham Heart Study

One line of evidence comes from people involved in the Framingham Heart Study, which dates back to the 1940s. Back then, very little was known about why people had heart attacks. This landmark study, which continues to this day, sought to answer that question. In 1948, researchers recruited more than fifty-two hundred men and women between the ages of 30 and 62 who were living in the Boston suburb of Framingham, Massachusetts. They recorded their height, weight, family health history, and gave them a physical exam every other year.

Over the years, scientists began collecting more data from the participants, such as measuring their blood pressure and cholesterol levels, and asking them about their eating, exercise, and smoking habits. In 1971, the Offspring Study, which includes the children (and their spouses) of the original group, was launched. And researchers began recruiting the third generation in 2002. Among the most important discoveries from the study was that cigarette smoking and obesity increase the risk of heart disease, and physical activity could lower that risk.

Researchers also found that over about a thirty-year period, the average participant gained about 20 pounds. This typical, slow gain is healthy and normal. The number of calories these participants ate balanced the number of calories they burned within a tiny percent during those years. If you figure that the average person eats about one million calories per year and you calculate the energy cost of those 20 pounds (that is, how many extra calories would a person have to eat each day, on average), it comes out to about 10 additional calories per day. That's less than The amount of calories in a single jelly bean! The body's internal control system is very is precise.

The Minnesota Starvation Study

Just a few years before the Framingham study began, a very different type of experiment was already underway in Minnesota, led by Ancel Keys. Dr. Keys is known for his pioneering work on the link between saturated fat and heart disease and for the development of K-rations, the balanced, portable meals given to soldiers during World War II. But his study involving a group of thirty-six conscientious objectors who volunteered to starve for the sake of science ranks as his most intriguing yet controversial work. Today, ethical regulations would never allow this type of study to take place.

The purpose of the study was to understand the physical and mental effects of starvation, anticipating the need to learn the best ways to re-feed people who had experienced extreme starvation (namely, civilians throughout Europe after World War II). The men endured six months of semistarvation, eating a diet similar to that in war-torn Europe—lots of potatoes and turnips and very little meat or dairy products. During the study, the men had to continue exercising, walking at least 22 miles a week, or about 3 miles a day. They were rationed about 1,600 calories per day—approximately three quarters of what these healthy young men needed to stay at their previously normal weight levels.

The men lost an average of about 25% of their body weight over six months, which caused them to resemble the concentration camp survivors they were hoping to help. They became sluggish, uncoordinated, depressed, and irritable. Keys documented the study in a two-volume tome, *The Biology of Human Starvation,* which includes this description penned by one volunteer:

> I'm hungry. I'm always hungry—not the hunger that comes when you miss lunch but a continual cry from the body for food. At times I can almost forget about it but there is nothing that can hold my interest for long.

These feelings may be familiar to veteran dieters who've tried very low-calorie diets. Even among people who are overweight or obese (unlike these normal-weight volunteers), the very same mechanisms kick in during the self-imposed starvation of a diet. Faced with the physical and emotional strain, the body fights back to stay alive. Keys calculated that the men's metabolic rates had decreased by about 40%

by the end of the starvation period. One volunteer said it was as if his "body flame [was] burning as low as possible to conserve precious fuel and still maintain [the] life process."

After six months of starvation, the men entered a rehabilitation phase, during which they gradually received increasing amounts of food over a three-month period. Perhaps not surprisingly, the men's response to this relative abundance provoked some unusual behaviors. Some ate until they vomited and then asked for more. Others ate until they weren't physically capable of eating another bite of food, yet they still claimed they were hungry. Again, these behaviors may sound familiar to people who've tried so-called crash diets designed for rapid weight loss.

The take-home lesson is that it's extremely challenging to try to lose a lot of weight over a short time period. Your body will rebel against these efforts, helping you regain the weight you've lost and possibly triggering strange (and potentially unhealthy) eating behaviors.

The Vermont Prison Overfeeding Study

Whereas the Keys study explored the body's response to a minimal number of calories, another intriguing study looked at the opposite end of the spectrum: calorie overload. In 1964, researchers at the Vermont College of Medicine asked volunteers to gain 15% to 25% of their body weight in less than three months.

The impetus for this study was to better understand exactly what happens to the body during weight gain. For instance, do fat cells increase in number or simply grow larger? At first, the scientists sought volunteers from a usually reliable source of guinea pigs: graduate and medical students at the college. But the study design, which required the volunteers to eat four large meals a day at the nutrition lab, proved far too time-consuming for busy students. So the researchers turned to a more captive crowd: inmates at the Vermont State Prison. They hired a cook to prepare the meals and served the food on china plates instead of tin. The prisoner's ample diets included standard American fare: cereal, eggs, and toast for breakfast, sandwiches for lunch, and dinners of meat, potatoes, and vegetables. The fourth meal, which the men ate just before bedtime, was similar to breakfast.

The volunteers started out at normal weights, which ranged from about 135 to 185 pounds. During the ten-week-long study, the men managed to gain between 15% and 25% of their body weight, which amounted to an average of nearly 36 pounds. To do so, they had to eat 8,000 to 10,000 calories a day—more than three times the normal number of calories they would have needed to maintain their weight. The weight changes were largely due to gains in body fat. By taking small samples of fat from the men's bellies, thighs, and arms before and after the overfeeding, the researchers demonstrated that this excess fat didn't create new fat cells but rather expanded the existing ones.

This study and similar ones on the prisoners revealed other interesting phenomena related to body weight and the set point. Researchers found that the prisoner's metabolic rates went into overdrive after the overfeeding period. These changes provide further evidence of the body's drive to restore balance and return to its set point. When the experiment ended and the men went back to eating regular amounts of food, they lost weight quite quickly—not just because they were eating less but because their metabolic rates were still racing. Note that the prisoners did not remain at the new, higher weights for very long, so they did not reset their set points to new, higher levels. That contrasts with people who have been overweight for long periods of time.

The rapid weight loss these prisoners experienced is the mirror image of what happens when overweight people try to lose weight. If your set point is too high and you try to lose weight quickly, your body will fight to defend that weight and slow down your metabolism. But if your set point is within a normal range, your metabolism will speed up when you gain weight quickly.

In recent years, many studies have reaffirmed the observations from these historic reports. One pivotal 1995 study, by Jules Hirsch and colleagues at the Rockefeller University in New York City, used sophisticated techniques to carefully measure the metabolic rates of forty-one obese and nonobese volunteers who followed strict diets that caused them to either lose or gain 10% of their body weight. The researchers found that when people gained 10% of their usual weight, their bodies focused less on conserving energy and more on wasting it. But when people lost more than 10% of their usual weight, the opposite occurred: their bodies fought to save energy rather than expend it. This explains why it's so difficult to lose more than 10% of your weight at a time.

So no matter where you start (overweight, thin, or somewhere in between) and no matter how you manipulate your diet (eating too much or too little), your metabolic rate will automatically adjust in an effort to keep you at the same set point.

Movie Stars

The set point phenomenon also explains why many actors manage to gain and lose relatively large amounts of weight for their movie roles. Although while you might think that getting paid to sit around and eat donuts all day sounds great, anecdotal evidence described in various media reports suggests otherwise. For example, Renée Zellweger, who gained 20 pounds for her role in the movie *Bridget Jones's Diary,* described her experience as "force feeding." According to one story, Zellweger gorged on pizza, candy bars, Fettuccine Alfredo, and peanut butter sandwiches and stopped working out. George Clooney, who gained about 35 pounds to play a CIA agent in *Syriana,* was reportedly depressed about not being able to exercise. Others actors have dropped large amounts of weight, such as Adrien Brody, who lost 30 pounds to portray a Holocaust survivor in *The Pianist.* His sparse diet, which consisted mainly of small amounts of protein and steamed vegetables, left him cranky. Tom Hanks not only lost 30 pounds for *Philadelphia* but later gained and then lost 50 pounds for *Cast Away.* These rebounds provide further support that the human body is able to return to its normal, healthy set point provided it doesn't stay at an elevated set point for too long.

External Forces Trump Inner Balance

You may be thinking if your body is so good at defending your set point, how did your set point become too high? Ultimately, your behavior—how you respond to the environment—trumps your physiology, or your body's inner workings. Eating is complex behavior that is affected by many different factors, including genetics. How food tastes, how hungry we feel, and even how we respond to social cues around food (for example, whether we eat more at a party or while alone) are all affected by our genes. And these genetic differences affect how we respond to our environment. Over the past few decades, changes in our society have altered our environment dramatically. Oversized portions of high-calorie (and often inexpensive) foods are readily available, day and night. And modern conveniences—everything from electric toothbrushes to leaf blowers to cars—mean we don't have as many opportunities to exercise. These and other factors, which are detailed

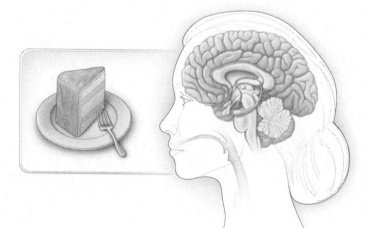

The cerebral cortex, or "cognitive" brain, is a thin layer of gray matter that cloaks the brain's cerebrum. The site of complex thought, your cortex processes the many environmental cues that drive you to eat—for example, the sight, smell, and taste of a piece of cake. The amygdala, the seat of your feelings and emotions, is the "emotional" brain. Together, your thoughts and feelings can override the controlled balance of your hypothalamus, or "metabolic" brain. That's why seeing and smelling a slice of cake—especially if you're feeling sad or worried—may prompt you to eat it, even if you're not hungry.

in the next chapter, are the driving forces behind our rising set points.

On a fundamental level, we eat to survive. Leptin and other hormones regulate this unconscious drive. But we also have a conscious desire to eat, which is clearly affected by the smell, taste, and appearance of foods. Your emotional state also comes into play. Some people eat more (or less) when they're upset, angry, or depressed (For more on breaking these patterns, see Chapter 9). We also eat out of habit, simply because it's time for lunch (or a snack or dinner) or because people around us are eating. As in most cultures, Americans often plan their work and social schedules around eating rituals.

Set Point Sabotage: Our Toxic Environment

The genetic background loads the gun, but the environment pulls the trigger.

—George Bray, M.D.,
    chief of clinical obesity,
    Pennington Biomedical Research Center,
    Baton Rouge, Louisiana

Food is cheaper now by a long way, more abundantly available, more highly refined and more pressingly sold to us by very clever advertising companies and techniques. The remarkable thing is how anybody stays thin.

—Andrew Prentice, Ph.D.,
    professor of international nutrition,
    London School of Hygiene and Tropical Medicine

You may think it's pretty obvious why people are overweight: they eat too much and exercise too little. Basically, that's true, but far too simplistic. As with many things in life, a multitude of factors often underlie a simple truth. A unique combination of influences—both internal and external—determine how much each person eats and exercises, and ultimately how much he or she weighs.

By internal influences, I'm talking about your genes, which orchestrate all of your body's biological functions, both physical and mental. External influences are all the things outside your body—your surroundings or environment. Both of these factors can affect your physiology (how your body functions) and your behavior (for example, what you put in your mouth and how much you exercise).

> ### Defining Overweight and Obese
>
> As the Framingham study showed, American adults gain on average about 20 pounds in middle age. Of course, there's a wide range, with some people gaining no weight and others gaining more than 20 pounds. People who gain about twice the average—that is, 40 pounds—fall into the overweight category. This corresponds to silhouette 4. But people who gain three times the average (60 pounds) are obese, which corresponds to silhouette 5 or higher. Doctors and researchers use a somewhat more precise measurement to determine overweight and obesity, called the body mass index, or BMI, explained in detail in Chapter 4.

By learning more about each of these influences and how they interact, I hope you'll better understand the roots of your own personal weight-related challenges. Some of these factors will be obvious, but some will be novel and may become the "aha moment" or "tipping point" that can spur you to move forward in your journey.

Although genetic factors are important, they don't explain the ballooning rates of overweight and obese people in the United States over the past thirty years. During that time, our genes haven't changed, but the environment certainly has. To a large extent, you can control your environment, which I will help you do in the later chapters of this book. First, let's explore how and why today's modern environment, combined with our ancient genetic legacy to survive, conspires to make gaining weight so easy and losing weight so hard.

GENETIC INFLUENCES

To date, more than four hundred genes are thought to be involved with weight control, with more being discovered every year. We all know of families (perhaps yours is one?) in which many members seem to gain weight very easily. Then there are other families that have similar eating patterns but remain slim. Or perhaps your sister is as thin as a rail, but you've always been pudgy, even though she seems to eat more than you.

In one pivotal study on the genetics of weight gain, researchers asked twelve pairs of identical twins (all young men) to eat 1,000 extra calories a day for nearly three months. As you'd expect, each twin pair, who share all their genetic material, responded quite similarly to the excess calories, gaining similar amounts of weight. But when comparing one set of twins to another, researchers saw wide variations in the men's weight gain, ranging from about 10 to 30 pounds. What's more, the men also differed in where on their bodies they tended to accumulate fat. For example, some twins were up to six times more likely to gain weight in their bellies than other twins. This tendency, which experts refer to as having an apple-shaped body, can raise the risk of diabetes, heart disease, and other health problems.

This study and others show that genes affect how much and where people tend to store fat and explain why kids tend to resemble their parents in terms of body size and shape. Experts believe these genes may affect resting energy expenditure, or the amount of calories you burn when you're at rest, as described in Chapter 1.

Favorite Foods

Genes may even influence what you choose to eat. Scientists at the Monell Chemical Senses Center in Philadelphia uncovered differences in a bitterness-sensing gene they say could explain why some kids turn up their noses at vegetables, many of which taste a bit bitter. Kids who were bitter-sensitive were also more likely to have a sweet tooth. Although the authors say these differences may account for what people tend to eat, they note that age also plays a role, since the children's mothers (despite having a similar genetic profile) tended to be less sensitive to bitterness than kids.

A fondness for salty french fries, cheesecake, and other fatty foods may also have a genetic basis. Studies suggest that overweight people tend to prefer fatty foods more than lean people. French scientists discovered a tongue taste receptor in rats that appears to detect fat. Interestingly, the receptor is a protein, CD36, involved in fat storage that's also found in other tissues throughout the body. When the researchers created genetically modified mice and rats that lacked the protein, the animals showed no preference for fatty foods. In contrast, normal animals clearly preferred fatty foods, and their digestive organs began cranking out fat-processing substances after researchers placed fatty acids on their tongues. That didn't happen with the gene-altered animals.

Eating Habits

Genes influence not only what you like to eat but also how hungry you feel ("perceived hunger") as well as how much and when you prefer to eat. For example, uncontrolled overeating is a practice known as disinhibition. The flip side is dietary restraint, or the practice of trying to curb your eating. Studies have shown that the latter and perceived hunger seem to be affected by genetic factors. Disinhibition, however, appears to be more strongly affected by a person's environment.

All in the Family

Studies of twins and of people who are adopted confirm that genes play a large role in whether a person will become overweight, accounting for perhaps as much as 80% of the risk. For instance, adopted people nearly always resemble their birth parents rather than their adoptive parents in terms of body size. If both of your parents are overweight, your risk is very high. If only one parent is, your risk is somewhat lower. Even having siblings or second-degree relatives (grandparents, aunts, uncles, nieces, or nephews) who are overweight will boost your chances. The age at which you became overweight is also telling: The younger you were when you became overweight, the higher your risk of being an overweight adult. If you were already carrying excess weight at age 10, the chances that you have a strong genetic tendency toward weight gain are much higher than if you didn't become over-

The Snickers Test

In case you're wondering how researchers determine how hungry or full a person feels, one tool they use is known as the Snickers test. The test involves eating a standard-size Snickers bar at 10:00 A.M. after an overnight fast. The person then records how hungry or full he or she feels, starting just before eating the candy bar and then every thirty minutes for the next three hours. The test uses a scale similar to the Hunger and Satiety Scale below, a 9-point scale with responses ranging from stuffed to starving. Snickers bars "really satisfy," as the ads say, not only because they're tasty and chewy, but because they contain the right mix of protein, carbohydrate, and fat to make you feel full.

Hunger and Satiety Scale

9 Starving, cranky, irritable
8 Very hungry
7 Hungry—ready to eat
6 Beginning hunger
5 Neither hungry nor full
4 Comfortably full
3 Very full
2 Uncomfortably full
1 Stuffed, feeling sick

You can do your own Snickers test at home, but try these variations: Eat the bar very slowly, over a period of twenty minutes. Notice how much more you enjoy it and how much more satisfied you feel than if you eat it quickly. (Better yet, try this with a bowl of cereal, fruit, and milk instead of a candy bar.)

The real purpose of showing you this scale is to make you aware of the ideal satiety zone, which is between 4 and 7. The idea is to train yourself to never eat so much that you're very full (a score of 3 or lower) but also never to let yourself get to the point where you're very hungry (8 or 9). Chapter 5 goes into more detail about this concept.

weight until age 20 or later. When you pile on pounds as an adult rather than as a child, environmental influences are probably more to blame than genetics.

In general, pinpointing genetic factors that cause obesity is difficult, because the effect of any one specific gene is likely to be small and will interact with environmental factors. And let me reemphasize that genetic factors only load the gun. Having a strong family history of overweight doesn't necessarily mean you will be (or become) overweight.

The Thrifty Gene Legacy

When it comes to genes, you probably think only of those that you inherited from your parents and grandparents. But the genetic legacy from your distant ancestors is also relevant. Thousands of years ago, our ancestors had to survive food-scarce migrations out of Africa or across the Bering Strait. To do this, they stored energy by eating as much as they could when food was plentiful. And to conserve this fuel, their body's internal calorie-burning process slowed down. Natural selection honed this survival mechanism over centuries. People who couldn't store fat to survive the lean times were less likely to live and pass on their genes. Today, 85% of us have thrifty genes—the genes that help conserve and hold on to excess weight. In effect, our bodies have been programmed not only to prefer fat but also to store and retain it.

Although our bodies have a built-in defense against starvation, the opposite isn't true. There is no internal brake that naturally prevents us from overeating. In fact, this phenomenon holds true for fluids as well as food. Marathon runners are more likely to die from drinking too much water (a condition called hyponatremia, caused by dangerously low sodium levels in the blood) than they are to die of dehydration. The powerful feeling of thirst propels them to drink, but there's not an equally strong sensation telling them to stop drinking water. These unconscious urges to drink and eat—and no urge to stop—are good examples of the body's tendency to protect itself in times of extreme deprivation.

TRENDS IN ADULT WEIGHT GAIN

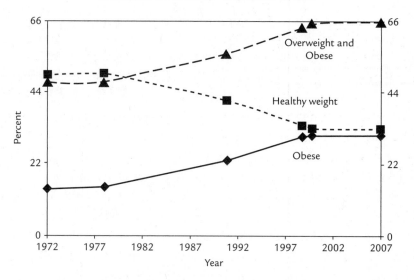

Compared to the 1970s, far more people are now overweight or obese, as this graph illustrates. (*"**Overweight**"* corresponds to silhouette 4 and *"**Obese**"* corresponds to silhouette 5 and higher.) News reports herald the discovery of genes linked to overweight and obesity, but genes alone can't explain such a rapid rise. The growing trend of excess weight among the entire U.S. population seems to be nearly universal, affecting all demographic groups, providing further evidence that changes in the environment are at the root of this epidemic. The good news is that the rise has stopped, as rates of overweight and obesity have leveled off in the past few years.

Sources: National Health and Nutrition Examination Survey (National Center for Health Statistics); *Cancer Trends Progress Report—2005 Update* (National Cancer Institute, 2005).

ENVIRONMENTAL INFLUENCES

Environment refers to all the conditions and circumstances that surround you throughout your life, starting at the moment of your conception. Here are some of the environmental factors related to body weight that come into play at different stages of your life.

Before Birth

Your surroundings can affect you even before you're born. Researchers sometimes call these in utero exposures fetal programming. Some research suggests that babies of mothers who smoked during pregnancy are more likely to become overweight as adults than babies of nonsmokers, even though smokers' babies tend to be smaller at birth. Although the reasons behind this phenomenon aren't fully understood, one hypothesis is that nicotine may affect the baby's developing brain, causing behavior changes that impact the child's impulse control and, in turn, appetite and food choices later in life. A similar phenomenon occurs in babies born to mothers who have diabetes. The mother's illness boosts levels of certain compounds that promote growth, which are transmitted to the developing fetus. Compared to babies born to healthy mothers, babies born to mothers with diabetes tend to weigh more at birth, and this excess weight may linger throughout life.

Early Childhood

Although many studies suggest that breast-feeding helps protect against obesity during childhood and adolescence, one large study found no difference in obesity rates among adult women who were bottle-fed as babies versus those who were breast-fed.

Once babies start eating solid food, healthy choices become more critical. But by early toddlerhood, or around 15 months, french fries are a toddler's most commonly eaten "vegetable," according to one report, which also found that some babies as young as 7 months have been given soda. Nearly a quarter of 19- to 24-month-olds don't eat any fruits and vegetables in a day, yet they eat sweets, desserts, or salty snacks at least once a day. Young children who eat fries and other high-calorie junk foods, including sugary sodas, develop a taste for these unhealthy foods, which can last for a lifetime. Many start watching television around this age, as well (see "The TV Trap" later in this chapter).

The School-Age Years

Even if parents manage to limit their children's exposure to junk food before they turn 5, once kids go to school, it's pretty tough to avoid the stuff. According to the Center for Science in the Public Interest (CSPI) in Washington, D.C., 83% of elementary schools, 97% of middle/junior high schools, and 99% of senior high schools sell foods out of vending machines, school stores, or à la carte. What are kids buying? Soft drinks, sports drinks, imitation fruit juices, chips, candy, cookies, and snack cakes (see the diagram). Fortunately, efforts are underway to make vending machine and school lunch offerings more healthy (see the Appendix).

SCHOOL VENDING MACHINE PYRAMID

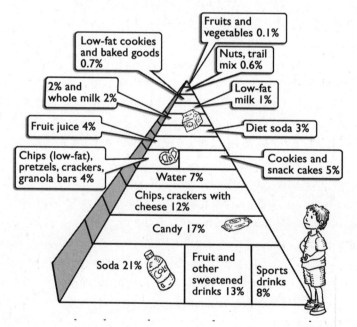

A 2003 study from CSPI had 120 volunteers in 24 states survey the contents of 1,420 vending machines in 251 middle, junior high, and high schools. In both middle and high schools, 75% of beverage options and 85% of snacks were what experts (and most people) consider junk food.

Source: Center for Science in the Public Interest (www.cspinet.org).

Not only do schools provide ready access to junk food, they also fail to include enough physical activity during the school day. Thirty percent of states don't require kids in elementary and middle school to take physical education classes. In 1991, 42% of students nationwide had a daily physical education class. In 2003, the percentage had dropped to 28%. And kids who watch a lot of television and play video games at home instead of being active may be programming themselves for a sedentary future.

Young Adulthood and Midlife

Your set point is first set when you stop growing, around age 18. Unless you are above a healthy weight at that time, you would (ideally) stay at that weight for the rest of your life. But as people move through their late teens and beyond, they're likely to experience a number of life changes that may affect their weight. One example is weight gain during the early college years, known as the freshman 15.

As people leave school and move into the workforce, they usually have less time for leisure activities, which may include organized sports or other exercise. That's especially true for those whose jobs require sitting at a computer most of the day, as is now increasingly common for many careers.

For women, pregnancy can be a challenge weight-wise. Although some women manage to lose their "baby weight," others find the extra pounds difficult to shed. Both women and men often find that the demands of parenthood lead to higher stress levels, less sleep, and less time to exercise, although some of these changes may be temporary. And some parents develop kid-food syndrome, eating macaroni and cheese, chicken nuggets, and other foods targeted at the younger set (more on this in Chapter 6).

Other major life events—marriage, divorce, or the death of a spouse, partner, family member, or close friend—often alter people's typical patterns, potentially causing them to eat more or exercise less, although the opposite may also be true. Of course, many of these events can occur throughout the adult years. The same is true for health-related causes of weight gain.

The Second 50 Years

As you grow older, everything slows down: You don't move quite as fast as when you were younger. Likewise, your body doesn't burn calories as quickly. A slower metabolism is often fingered as the cause of middle-age spread, but a tendency to exercise less may also be partly to blame. Despite the widespread notion that menopause often leads to weight gain, studies suggest it's not the hormonal changes that trigger weight gain but the concurrent slowed metabolism and decreased exercise that often happen around the same time.

A problem that sometimes parallels the freshman 15 is known as empty nest syndrome, which can strike parents when their kids leave home. Mom and Dad gain weight because they don't scale down their shopping and cooking, which leaves them excess food to nosh on. Another common challenge is a job that requires you to eat away from home a great deal, whether you're traveling or attending business lunches or dinners.

With age also comes a greater likelihood of developing a chronic disease. Those that affect your metabolism, such as type 2 diabetes or thyroid disease, affect your weight. Other serious illnesses—heart disease, stroke, arthritis, or cancer—can too. For instance, the disease may leave you too weak, tired, or otherwise unable to exercise. A knee or hip replacement, or a broken bone or other injury, can make exercise impossible or difficult, at least temporarily. Certain medications can lead to weight gain, either by increasing appetite or slowing metabolism. (See the Appendix for more information on these drugs.)

Smoking, Drinking, and Other Addictive Behaviors

People who smoke cigarettes tend to be leaner than those who don't. Smokers (especially women) often worry that they'll gain weight after quitting. While that's not necessarily a given, some experts suggest that the lower smoking rates among Americans have contributed to rising obesity rates. Of course, no one would ever recommend smoking as a weight-loss aid. The benefits of quitting smoking far outweigh the risks (and expense) of staying addicted. But it's worth noting that kicking the habit may pose yet another challenge to your weight-loss efforts.

Unlike smoking, drinking alcohol may offer some health benefits, but only in moderation. You've undoubtedly heard that moderate drinking—defined as a drink a day for women and two drinks a day for men—can help prevent heart disease. But if you don't already drink alcohol, there's no reason to start to protect your heart, as there are plenty of alternative strategies, such as the healthy eating and exercise habits described in this book.

If you enjoy drinking alcohol, fine. A glass of wine sipped with a meal is one thing; downing two gin and tonics before dinner is another. The problem with cocktail hour is that your cheery, inebriated self is less likely to stick to a healthy eating plan during dinner. In fact, alcohol is a very common trigger for disinhibition. And alcoholic beverages have a lot of calories (around 100 to 150 calories per drink), which can change your set point 10 to 15 pounds if you drink daily.

Note that quitting any addictive substance—tobacco, drugs, alcohol, and so on—can cause weight gain. This may happen because people seek pleasure from food instead of from the other substances.

THE BIG TWO: TOO MUCH FOOD AND NOT ENOUGH EXERCISE

In addition to the unique life circumstances that shape each person's environment, American society as a whole represents a powerful environmental influence on all of us. These days, we don't burn calories harvesting or hunting food as our ancestors did. Instead, we simply stroll into restaurants, where oversized portions of high-calorie (and often inexpensive) foods are readily available, day and night. Just as the risk of lung cancer rises with exposure to toxic cigarette smoke, the risk of overweight and obesity balloons with exposure to this toxic food environment.

Number 1: Too Much Food

According to the Centers for Disease Control and Prevention (CDC) in Atlanta, Americans are eating more calories on average than they did thirty years ago. Between 1971 and 2000, the average man added 168 calories to his daily fare, while the average woman added 335 calories a day. Even if that doesn't sound like much, it adds up over time.

Many factors have paved the way to this calorie excess. For one thing, food is less expensive than it was thirty years ago. In 1970, Americans spent about 15% of their disposable income on food, whereas in 2004, we spent about 11%.

But we're spending far more of those food dollars on away-from-home foods—that is, foods purchased at restaurants, snack bars, cafeterias, and so forth, as opposed to supermarkets or convenience stores. In fact, the percentage of money spent on away-from-home food nearly doubled, from 26% in 1970 to 46% in 2004. Not surprisingly, the number of food service establishments also nearly doubled during that same time period.

What's so bad about these trends? People who eat out more are more likely to be obese and to have more body fat. Research shows that women who eat out more than five times a week eat about 290 more calories on average each day than women who eat out less often. Also, most of these restaurant visits—up to 75%—are to fast-food joints. Using drive-through or curbside service at these restaurants is becoming more common, too—which means not only are people eating more high-calorie fast food, they're burning even fewer calories to get it!

In the 1970s, dining out accounted for . . .	In 2004, dining out accounted for . . .
26.3% of total food expenditures	46% of total food expenditures
16% of all meals and snacks	27% of all meals and snacks
18% of total caloric intake	34% of total caloric intake
18% of total fat intake	38% of total fat intake

Source: FDA Keystone Forum Reports on Away-from-Home Foods.

Too Much of a Bad Thing

The problem with eating out is simple: it encourages people to eat too much high-calorie food. We've all seen how portion sizes in fast-food restaurants have ballooned in recent years, as the movie *Super Size Me* helped illuminate. In the 1950s, fast-food restaurants offered one serving size. Today, a typical portion of french fries from McDonald's contains three times more calories than when the franchise began. The burger giant actually phased out its Super Size menu by the end of 2004, but the practice of offering larger portion sizes for just a fraction more of the cost of the "regular" size remains popular at many fast-food franchises.

And oversized servings (a trend known as portion distortion) are everywhere, from convenience store Big Gulps the size of small buckets to sit-down restaurants that serve individual plates of pasta large enough to feed a family of four. In many restaurants, portion sizes of both food and drink are twice as big or more than standard serving sizes defined by the Food and Drug Administration (FDA).

People tend to eat what's in front of them, even after they're full. In one study, twenty-three normal-weight and overweight adults were recruited to eat at a nutrition lab for two 11-day periods. During one period, they were served standard-sized portions. But during the second period, the portion size was bumped up by 50%. The volunteers ate an average of 400 more calories a day when served these hefty portions, which added up to a total of 4,473 more calories over 11 days. In theory, that could add 1¼ pounds to the average person—in less than two weeks. You might assume that people cut back during other meals after overeating, but research shows that's not usually the case.

When people buy prepackaged foods, like a giant cookie or soda, they tend to finish the whole thing, sometimes even if it doesn't taste good! One study documented this phenomenon with popcorn in a movie theater (the bigger the tub, the more people ate)—even though the popcorn was stale.

People like large portion sizes because they feel as though they're getting a bargain. Buffet and all-you-can-eat restaurants are another good example of this troubling trend. Even if you don't frequent such restaurants, you've probably been to a potluck where the wide array of tempting choices led you to eat more than you should—yet another trend that's been observed by researchers.

Junk Food, Junk Food Everywhere

It's hardly surprising that Americans get one-third of their calories from junk food. Soft drinks, salty snacks, and candy are far more readily available than lower-calorie choices like salads and whole fruits. You can buy snacks or meals at shopping centers, sports stadiums, movie theaters, roadside rest stops, twenty-four-hour convenience stores, even gyms and health clubs. Vending machines featuring candy, chips, and soda aren't just in schools but in workplaces, libraries, swimming pools, bowling alleys—you name it. Knowing that these convenient snacks are just a short walk away means that many people won't bother to bring a healthier snack from home.

You might think that it's the fat content of many of these foods that's the root of the problem. Not necessarily. In fact, research shows that the fat content of our diet has actually gone down in the last twenty-five years. But many low-fat foods are very high in calories because they contain large amounts of sugar to improve their taste and palatability. Many low-fat foods are actually equivalent to or higher in calories than foods that are not low-fat.

CALORIE COMPARISONS

Fat-Free or Reduced-Fat	Calories	Regular	Calories
Peanut butter, 2 T	187	Peanut butter, 2 T	191
Chocolate chip cookies, 3 small cookies	118	Chocolate chip cookies, 3 small cookies	142
Nonfat vanilla frozen yogurt, ½ cup	100	Whole-milk vanilla frozen yogurt, ½ cup	104
Light vanilla ice cream, 7% fat, ½ cup	111	Vanilla ice cream, 11% fat, ½ cup	133
Low-fat blueberry muffin, 1 small (2½ inches)	131	Blueberry muffin, 1 small (2½ inches)	138
Baked tortilla chips, 1 oz.	113	Tortilla chips, 1 oz.	143

Low-fat foods contain large amounts of sugar and other additives so that they taste (and feel) better in your mouth. Contrary to popular belief, many low-fat foods actually contain as many or more calories as their higher-fat counterparts.

Source: National Heart, Lung, and Blood Institute.

The TV Trap

Even when you're not around food, you're exposed to advertisements for food—mainly on TV, which the average American watches more than four hours per day. The latest data from the National Health and

Nutrition Examination Survey revealed that people with overweight and obesity spend more time watching television and playing video games than people of normal weight. Watching television more than two hours a day also raises the risk of becoming overweight in children, even in those as young as three years old. We should be concerned that about a third of children age 6 and under have a TV in their bedroom and that just over half of all kids between the ages of 8 and 16 do.

Contrary to what you might think, the problem isn't so much that watching TV takes the place of exercising or doing other activities that burn more calories (although sitting in front of the tube burns only slightly more calories than sleeping and less than other sedentary pursuits such as sewing or reading). Food advertisements appear to play a big role. The average hour-long TV show features about eleven food and beverage commercials, all of which are designed to encourage people to eat. During Saturday morning cartoons, kids see an average of one commercial every five minutes, most of which feature high-sugar cereals, candy bars, and other junk food. Kids younger than 8 can't distinguish between advertising and regular programming, so they're especially vulnerable to these messages. And advertisers often rely on familiar cartoon or movie characters to peddle their products. More healthful, lower-calorie options like fruits and salads are scarce, both on TV and in real life.

With all these advertisements and the distraction of the TV, it shouldn't be a surprise that studies show that eating food in front of the TV stimulates people to eat more calories, especially more calories from fat. In fact, a study that limited the amount of TV kids watched found that it helped them lose weight, but not because they became more active. The difference was that they ate fewer snacks, which children ate when they were watching television but not when doing other (even sedentary) activities.

While TV commercials make up the lion's share of restaurant advertising, food ads appear in many other places, including magazines, newspapers, billboards, and on the Internet. We're also exposed to restaurant and food ads through coupons, email, text messaging, or viral marketing, which refers to a strategy that relies on the tell-a-friend technique, either in person or online. Product placements, like a can of soda in a TV show or movie, are yet another way people are subtly urged to eat and drink certain products.

The Constant Grazer

The ubiquitous reminders and availability of food foster other problems. People tend to snack more, which causes them to lose their hunger cues. That's a problem because instead of eating when you're actually hungry, you put food into your mouth just because it's there. Many people also eat when they are thirsty, because the thirst response isn't as strong as the hunger response. That's why you should drink a glass of water when you think you're hungry and then wait fifteen minutes to decide if you still want to eat.

Food availability and the time crunch have led to a new eating etiquette, which has made eating in public—while walking, driving, or commuting, for example—commonplace. A related trend is the working lunch, or even the working dinner, whether at a desk or at a meeting. This can cultivate mindless eating or stress-related eating both of which can cause you to eat more calories than you need or want.

Some researchers think that the very act of eating irregularly, frequently, and on the run may contribute to obesity. Studies indicate that the brain's biological clock—the pacemaker that controls numerous other daily rhythms in the body—may help to regulate hunger and satiety signals. Ideally, these signals should keep our weight steady. They should prompt us to eat when our body fat falls below a certain level or when we need more body fat (during pregnancy, for example), and they should tell us when we feel full and should stop eating. Close connections between the brain's pacemaker and the appetite control center in the hypothalamus suggest that hunger and satiety are affected by time cues. Irregular eating patterns may disrupt the effectiveness of these cues in a way that promotes obesity.

Number 2: Not Enough Exercise

The government currently recommends thirty minutes of moderate exercise a day at least five days a week. Fewer than 25% of Americans meet that goal, but more people are exercising than in the late 1980s. At that time, nearly a third of people said they did no physical activity during their leisure time (such as walking, golfing, or gardening). By 2002, only a quarter of people said they did no physical activity.

Our daily lives don't offer many opportunities for activity. As already noted, children don't exercise as much in school, often because of cutbacks in physical education classes. Many people drive to work and spend much of the day sitting at a computer terminal. Because of the pressure to work long hours, many have trouble finding the time to go to the gym, play a sport, or exercise in other ways.

Lack of time isn't the only excuse for not exercising. According to an informal poll from the American Council on Exercise, many people feel too intimidated to go to a health club or gym. They're either self-conscious about how they look or are worried that they're too out of shape. Another common problem is not knowing how to use the equipment and feeling uncomfortable asking questions about how to use it. Many also complain that health clubs are too crowded or that the other patrons are rude.

People who don't like gyms have many other options, of course. But certain environmental circumstances can make these options challenging as well. For instance, it's difficult to walk outdoors in extreme weather conditions. In densely populated urban areas, people rely less on their cars and tend to walk more—to work, school, public transportation, stores, and other venues. People who live in suburban neighborhoods, however, don't have that option. In these areas, which planners describe as urban sprawl, nothing is within easy walking distance of anything else, so people spend much more time in their cars. The lack of sidewalks in many neighborhoods is another barrier. In fact, research shows that people living in sprawling counties tend to walk less in their leisure time, to weigh more, and are more likely to have high blood pressure.

Behavior-Related Influences

Clearly, our environment has made it much easier to eat more and exercise less, but what are the underlying reasons for these changes? In many families, both parents work, which makes it harder to find time to shop, prepare, and eat healthy foods together. Single-parent families have an added burden in this regard. After a long day at work, it's far easier to let kids watch television and order a take-out pizza.

Time pressures—whether for school, work, or family obligations—often lead people to eat on the run and to sacrifice sleep, both of which can contribute to weight gain. Research shows that the less you sleep, the more likely you are to gain weight. Lack of sufficient sleep tends to disrupt hormones that control hunger and appetite. In a 2004 study of more than a thousand volunteers, researchers found that people who slept less than eight hours a night had higher levels of body fat than those who slept more. People who slept the fewest hours weighed the most. (For more details, see Chapter 8.)

Stress and lack of sleep are closely connected to psychological well-being, which can affect diet and appetite, as anyone who's ever gorged on cookies or potato chips when feeling anxious or sad can attest. Some people eat more when they're affected by depression, anxiety, or other emotional disorders. In turn, overweight and obesity themselves can promote emotional disorders. If you repeatedly try to lose weight and fail, or if you succeed in losing weight only to gain it all back, the struggle can cause tremendous frustration over time, which can cause or worsen anxiety and depression, creating a vicious cycle.

Other psychological and social factors play a large role in how people eat, both at home and at restaurants. Many people eat calorie-laden comfort foods, like mashed potatoes or rich desserts, not to combat stress but out of nostalgia or familiarity. Holiday celebrations are another common cause of overindulgence, from the Thanksgiving feast to candy-centered holidays like Valentine's Day and Halloween.

THREE

The 10% Solution

For patients who are unable to attain and maintain substantial weight reduction, modest weight loss should be recommended; even a small amount of weight loss appears to benefit a substantial subset of obese patients.

—David J. Goldstein,
formerly of Lilly Research Laboratories,
Eli Lilly and Company and the Indiana
University of Medicine, Indianapolis, Indiana

B y now, you should have a better idea of exactly why losing weight can be challenging and why gaining weight is relatively easy. But weight loss doesn't have to be difficult. It's hard to make lasting changes if you fight against your set point by trying to lose too much weight too quickly. Instead, you need to work with your set point. Losing 10% of your body weight in a gradual fashion and then maintaining that loss for at least three to six months is the secret to resetting your set point.

FORGET FAD DIETS

Chances are you've already tried one or more of the many fad diets. These include everything from the one-food wonder diets, like the cabbage soup or grapefruit diet, to the fasting regimen promoted in the Master Cleanse diet, to the more complex regimens such as the Atkins, Zone, or Shangri-La diets. The problem is that none of these diet plans have any staying power for more than a few months. Fad diets don't give you the tools you need to lose weight and keep it off. It's just not reasonable to think you can stay on a restricted diet that omits an entire food group for the rest of your life. Following a fad diet inevitably means a slide back to your old eating habits, because you never learn to make permanent, healthful choices as you do in the set point solution. As a result, once you stop dieting, you quickly regain the pounds.

Americans seem to be wising up to this reality, according to a 2006 poll by America On the Move, a nonprofit group devoted to promoting healthful habits. More than two-thirds of the respondents said they're less likely to try a fad diet today compared to five years ago. Most had tried to lose weight at least once during the past five years, but 65% of these people said their efforts had failed.

The other big problem with fad diets is that they encourage you to lose too much weight too fast. Scientific evidence supports losing no more than 10% of your body weight at a time. The very first evidence for the 10% figure comes straight from my own work, dating back to my Ph.D. research at the Massachusetts Institute of Technology (MIT) in the early 1970s. We carried out controlled trials that randomly assigned people to different types of diets: very low-calorie diets that provided about 400 to 800 calories per day or balanced-deficit diets that provided the same number of calories as the person's usual diet minus 500 calories. People who lost weight rapidly on the very low-calorie diets regained more than half of all the weight they'd lost within two years. In contrast, those who followed a balanced-deficit diet lost 10% of their weight. But because they only regained small amounts of that weight over the next one to two years, they ended up losing as much or more as the very low-calorie group.

It turns out that the body's set point and its many regulatory hormones dictate the effectiveness of the 10% loss. That's the amount of weight you can lose before your body starts to fight back. Many clinical studies have confirmed this phenomenon. Of course, some people can lose more than 10% at a time, but few can then maintain that loss.

Seduced by Supplements?

Like many people trying to lose weight, you've no doubt wondered whether any of the widely advertised weight-loss supplements are worth trying. Perhaps you've even plunked down $30 for a bottle of the latest fat burner or hunger buster that's supposed to melt away pounds. If so, you're not alone: Americans spend an estimated $1.3 billion each year on these over-the-counter (OTC) products. More than twice as many people take these products than prescription weight-loss drugs, according to a 2006 survey.

What's wrong with this picture? For starters, the Food and Drug Administration (FDA) does not regulate these OTC products, contrary to widespread belief. Because they are neither food nor drugs, weight-loss aids are classified as dietary supplements, a category developed in 1994 under the Dietary Supplement Health and Education Act. As a result, individual nutrients (vitamins and minerals), herbs, and other plants with supposed medicinal value (phytomedicinals) can be sold without being tested for effectiveness or safety, provided they don't make any direct health or therapeutic claims. But they can make indirect claims, which have led to many unfounded assertions on labels and advertisements. These claims create confusion and unrealistic expectations for weight loss, not to mention a sense of despair and hopelessness among people who try the products. This can delay or derail efforts that actually do make a difference, like eating less and being physically active.

Safety is another concern. Manufacturers of these products aren't required to follow strict quality-control procedures, so products may contain much more or much less of the alleged active ingredients. In effect, you're using these products at your own risk. At best, all you'll have lost is some money. At worst, you could lose your life or develop a serious side effect such as a heart attack or stroke. That's what happened to a number of people who took ephedra *(Ma huang)*, a Chinese herb widely promoted for weight

(continued)

loss and boosting energy. The government documented ninety-two serious events caused by ephedra, including heart attack, stroke, seizures, and death. Although the FDA subsequently banned the sale of ephedra in 2004, the agency can't take a product off the market unless it's found to be dangerous. And because the FDA can't test every one of the thousands of supplements on the market, most will not be banned. In fact, supplements containing ephedra-like compounds (such as ephedrine, norephedrine, and methylephedrine) remain widely available, often in combination with other stimulants such as caffeine. The bottom line: don't waste your money or faith on dietary supplements for weight loss.

AVOID THE REBOUND

Think of your weight as being like a rubber band. If you stretch it gradually, there's a certain amount of give. But if you stretch it too hard or too fast, it can bounce right back or even snap. The faster and more drastically you try to lose weight, the more your body will want to return to its set point by regaining any lost weight (and sometimes more).

This is what your body is designed to do, after all. As I mentioned in Chapter 2, the human body has evolved to protect itself against starvation. And if you try to lose too much too fast, your body goes into starvation mode, slowing your metabolism and resisting weight loss in an effort to conserve the calories you do consume.

Until recently, the standard party line on weight loss was that only about 25% of people who try to lose weight actually do, and only 5% of those people manage to keep off the lost weight. With those dismal statistics, it's a wonder anyone even tries. But since the late 1980s, after I first published studies showing the benefits of a 10% weight loss, experts have gradually changed the way they think about dieting. Now, health professionals, government agencies, professional societies, and expert panels routinely recommend people to work toward gradual, more modest weight loss.

Is Yo-Yo Dieting a No-No?

Contrary to what some people think, yo-yo dieting (when your weight goes up and down, up and down) doesn't have any lasting effect on your body. Some early reports suggested that yo-yo dieting had negative health effects, which discouraged people from trying to lose weight, since they feared that yo-yo dieting was more harmful than staying overweight. Some patients say to me, "I can't lose any more weight. I've yo-yo dieted for years. People tell me my metabolism won't ever recover." That simply isn't true. Additional studies failed to find any link between yo-yo dieting and future health problems. Instead, staying overweight leads to future health problems. Losing weight is sort of like quitting smoking. Successful quitters often try a few times before they actually kick the habit. Giving up an unhealthy lifestyle can be equally challenging, so it's okay if you've tried a few diets that didn't work. In fact, there's not one thing in life that doesn't improve with practice.

THE POWER OF 10

To reset your set point, you need to lose 10% of your weight. Fortunately, that's very simple to calculate. For example, if you weigh 150 pounds, your goal would be to lose 15 pounds; if you weigh 220, your goal would be a 22-pound loss.

Many people who've struggled to lose weight have unrealistic goals of how much they can or should lose. For instance, a 45-year-old woman who is 5'3" and weighs 160 pounds may hope to lose 35 pounds. But she should first set a more manageable goal of losing just 16 pounds. Often, when I first mention the 10% rule, people smile and say, "Oh, I can do that!"

As a first step, I advise my patients to cut back on how much they eat by about 10% and to lose no more than 1 pound per week. (Chapter 5 is all about the strategies to accomplish this.) They need to stick with the plan until they've lost 10%. That may take anywhere from six months to a year or longer, which may sound frustratingly slow. Trust me—it's much more efficient in the long run. A slow, gradual approach that resets your set point will help protect against hunger and the need to drastically cut back on how much you eat, as well as help you avoid regaining weight. Keep in mind that it took a relatively long time for you to gain your excess weight. It's only natural that it will take a while to lose it.

Estimate how many calories you eat to maintain your current weight. If you are reasonably active, multiply your weight by 15 to find this number. For example, if you weigh 180 pounds, you eat approximately 2,700 calories a day. Cutting 10% means eating about 270 fewer calories per day (roughly the amount in a Snickers bar). But I'm actually

10% CALORIE CHART

If you are . . .	You eat about . . .	so	Cutting 10%, or . . .	will help you lose . . .
140 pounds	2,100 calories/day		210 calories/day	14 pounds
150	2,250		225	15
160	2,400		240	16
170	2,550		255	17
180	2,700		270	18
190	2,850		285	19
200	3,000		300	20
210	3,150		315	21
220	3,300		330	22
230	3,450		345	23
240	3,600		360	24
250	3,750		375	25
260	3,900		390	26

not a big advocate of counting calories. I feel it makes the whole process unnecessarily complicated. Besides, the reality is that no one, even experienced dietitians, can count calories with any degree of accuracy. (Chapter 5 details a study that proves this assertion—see "Calorie Confusion".) For those of you who are tuned in to calories, you may find the 10% chart helpful. But I'd like to stress that you don't need to worry about counting calories. Instead, I'll teach you a number of simple tricks to eat less. And to make sure you're staying on track, there's one crucial step you need to take every single day: the one you take onto your scale, as you'll read about in Chapters 4 and 10.

HOLDING STEADY

Once you reach your goal of losing 10%, you'll need to stick with your new, healthful habits, resisting the temptation to fall back into your old ways. If you're on a roll and can keep losing weight, that's great—you probably haven't stretched your inner rubber band as far as it will go. But most people will start to feel the pull after 5%. Some may be on the verge of snapping after losing 7% to 8%, while others may be able to go a bit beyond 10%. The key goal is not to give up the initial 7% to 10% weight loss for at least six months. The cycle can be repeated for additional weight loss after you've kept the pounds off for at least six months. This stepwise approach is crucial to achieving and maintaining a healthy weight for life.

People are more likely to be successful over the long term if they devote time to a holistic lifestyle plan than prevents weight regain, which includes eating quality food, being physically active, and sleeping seven to eight hours a night. All of these changes require careful time management, which is explained in greater detail in Chapter 8. Another helpful prescription is doing things that bring you pleasure that don't involve food, as described in Chapter 9. Find ways to relieve stress that make you feel good (talking with a friend, doing a relaxing hobby, or getting a massage, for example), you'll be less likely to turn to food for comfort.

By holding your weight at a steady level without losing additional weight, you will benefit by accepting and embracing the plateau period. This phase can be a bit frustrating for several reasons. First, you may feel discouraged because you don't get that same thrill of seeing the numbers on the scale inching downward. You may feel as though you've failed because you've hit the wall and stopped losing. At this point, it's tempting to throw up your hands and say, "I give up. I might as well go back to having ice cream for breakfast!" But instead of feeling defeated, you should celebrate the fact that you've reached your new set point. The wall or plateau is your body's way of telling you that it's had enough for now. You've rebalanced your body at a new lower weight. Now, give it some time to get readjusted and take time to appreciate all the improvements in your quality of life. If you've ever lost 10 or 20 pounds, you know that you can see and feel the difference.

The second challenge is that it's very tempting to slide back into old habits at this stage of the game. You may say, "I've been so good, I can eat this whole dessert!" Instead, you need to stay the course, reinforcing and making permanent the new lower-calorie, more healthful eating pattern that helped you reach your goal. In effect, your body's fuel efficiency standards have improved: instead of running like a V-6 engine, your body now resembles a more streamlined, efficient 4-cylinder engine. That's a positive change, because people with more fuel-efficient bodies live longer.

After you maintain your new, lower weight for six months, you can repeat the cycle and reset your set point again by losing another 10%. Through small, gradual changes in your daily habits, you'll be able to stay at that new, lower weight for the rest of your life. This prescription is vital to outsmarting the body's natural tendencies to regain weight.

Your body will want to hover at its new set point after the 10% weight loss. Many published studies confirm this tendency. Take charge of your new healthful lifestyle. Make every day a structured day by allocating enough time to eat, exercise, and get plenty of sleep.

EMBRACING THE PLATEAU

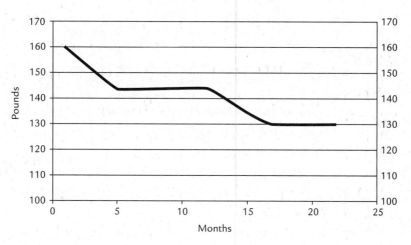

If you can lose 10% of your weight and maintain the loss for six months, (as in this example of Mary, who went from 160 to 144 pounds), you'll boost your chances of losing another 10%. Mary, whose story appears in Chapter 5, dropped from a silhouette 4 down to a silhouette 2 (see page 77) within two years. Think of the plateau as a time to rebuild your stamina and get your second wind before moving on to the second 10%.

THE BENEFITS OF 10%

You might think losing 10% of your weight won't really make that big a difference. Believe me, you'll be taking a very important step toward becoming (or staying) healthier and living longer.

Physical Appearance

You'll notice a difference in the way you look even after losing just a few pounds. You typically check your face in a mirror several times a day, so it's easy to see the weight loss from your face and neck, where it usually first becomes apparent. Most of us tend to lose weight from the top down, starting with the face and neck and moving to the chest, belly, hips, and finally the thighs. People who are more pear shaped (meaning they tend to carry most of their excess weight in their hips and thighs) may notice weight loss in their lower body first, since their upper body might be fairly slender.

To get a better sense of what a pound of fat looks like, the next time you're in the grocery store, stroll down the dairy aisle and pick up a pound of butter. Grab another one and imagine those 2 pounds on your chest, belly, or hips. You'd definitely notice the difference if you added those to your body—and you'll also see (and feel) the difference if you lose that same amount of weight. And that's just 2 pounds! Now imagine a bag filled with 12 pounds of butter. Think what it would be like to carry those 12 pounds around with you all day long—when you're getting dressed in the morning, taking a walk, working, shopping, running errands—whatever. You are probably already carrying at least that much excess weight on your body. But within just three months, you could lose those 12 pounds for good and be well on your way to resetting your set point.

Energy and Well-being

Looking better means feeling better. You'll see the benefits every time you look in the mirror. You'll also notice that you have more energy and your body will feel better overall. For instance, people often say their joints don't ache as much after they lose a little weight. Things that used to take a bit of effort, like walking up a flight of stairs, carrying groceries in from the car, or chasing after a small child, will be a bit easier after you've lightened your load. You'll start to sleep better. Just imagine waking up feeling rested instead of exhausted.

Health Benefits

This is the big one. We've known for more than half a century that excess weight can shorten a person's life span. Years ago, experts believed that eliminating health risks of these meant that you had to lose all of your excess weight. This was the impetus behind very low-calorie diets, in which people were essentially put on starvation diets and given only about 800 calories per day. These people were eager to return to a normal weight, so they were motivated to try to lose a lot of weight quickly. But, as you know by now, that's a recipe for disaster, triggering a rubber-band rebound of weight regain.

We now know that most of the health benefits of weight loss actually occur in the first 5% to 10% of weight loss. For example, I led a study that compared low-calorie and very low calorie diets in 187 people with obesity and high blood pressure. The study participants were supervised during a six-month diet period and a six-month maintenance period, then checked again after one year. Both groups had lost and then regained some of that lost weight, but they lost about 5% of their weight overall. Even with this modest loss, their diastolic blood pressure (the second number in a blood pressure measurement) dropped by 12 to 13 points, on average. Since then, many additional studies have confirmed this phenomenon with high blood pressure and other health conditions.

(Answers to the quizzes on the following pages are found on page 51.)

HIGH BLOOD PRESSURE

Test Your Knowledge #1

The percentage increase in high blood pressure among women who have gained an unhealthy amount of body weight compared to healthy-weight women is:

a. 5%
b. 16%
c. 50%
d. 23%

High blood pressure is about six times more common in people who have obesity than in those who are lean. For every pound you gain, your blood pressure rises an incremental amount. Research suggests that 22 pounds of excess weight can raise your systolic blood pressure (the first number in a blood pressure reading) by an average of 3 mm Hg and your diastolic blood pressure (the second number) by an average of 2.3 mm Hg. These increases translate into a 12% increased risk of heart disease and a 24% increased risk of stroke, according to a 2006 statement from the American Heart Association.

Luckily, the reverse also holds true; more than forty-five different trials show that losing weight can lower blood pressure, and in many cases, losing just small amounts of weight make a noticeable difference. In fact, for most people who are just beginning to develop high blood pressure (higher than 140/85), a 10-pound weight loss is the only treatment they'll need. For example, in one study, people who lost 10 pounds over six months reduced their systolic blood pressure by 2.8 mm Hg and their diastolic blood pressure by 2.5 mm Hg. These reductions in blood pressure were equal to the reductions brought about by treatment with blood pressure medications. Weight loss is so effective that many people with high blood pressure can stop taking blood pressure medicine after they lose weight, for as long as they are able to keep the weight off.

BLOOD LIPIDS (FATS)

Test Your Knowledge #2

A 10-to-20-pound weight gain increases women's risk of heart disease by:

a.　125%
b.　50%
c.　Less than 10%
d.　Not at all

Excess weight leads to an unfavorable level of blood lipids (cholesterol and triglycerides), which are another harbinger of heart disease and stroke. These diseases rank as the first and third leading causes of death in the United States, respectively. Specifically, people who are overweight tend to have higher levels of LDL ("bad") cholesterol and triglycerides and lower levels of HDL ("good") cholesterol. Several studies confirm that weight loss can improve these values by increasing HDL and lowering triglyceride levels, and (to a lesser extent) by lowering both total and LDL cholesterol.

DIABETES

Test Your Knowledge #3

Gaining 11 to 18 pounds increases a person's risk of developing type 2 diabetes by:

a. 0%
b. 50%
c. 200%
d. 400%

Type 2 diabetes, currently the nation's sixth leading cause of death, is so closely linked with overweight and obesity that we now use the term *diabesity* to describe the phenomenon. About 90% of people with type 2 diabetes are overweight or have obesity.

Obesity raises the risk of developing diabetes twenty-fold. Untreated or poorly controlled diabetes can lead to kidney failure, blindness, and foot or leg amputations. Numerous studies show that losing weight can help lower blood sugar levels, a hallmark of type 2 diabetes. A major trial of more than thirty-two hundred people who were at risk for developing type 2 diabetes found that people who lost just 7% of their weight and exercised about thirty minutes a day cut their risk of diabetes by 58%—more than participants who took metformin, a commonly prescribed medication for diabetes.

CANCER

Test Your Knowledge #4

On average, the estimated percentage of all cancer deaths in women accounted for by obesity is:

a. 5%
b. 10%
c. 20%
d. 30%

Did you know that obesity is second only to cigarette smoking as a cause of cancer death? According to an American Cancer Society study, obesity may account for 14% of all cancer deaths in men and 20% of all cancer deaths in women. In both men and women, a higher body mass index (BMI) was associated with a higher risk of dying from cancer of the esophagus, colon and rectum, liver, gallbladder, pancreas, or kidney. (BMI is a measure of body size based on height and weight. It is used by health care providers to determine whether a person is a normal weight, overweight, or obese. For more details and to calculate your own BMI, see Chapter 4.) In men, excess weight also increased the risk of dying from stomach or prostate cancer. In women, deaths from breast, uterine, cervical, or ovarian cancer were higher in women with higher BMIs.

Because cancer takes so long to develop, it's difficult to prove that losing weight can lower cancer risk. However, I coauthored a 2006 study that examined the effect of a low-fat diet in preventing breast cancer recurrence in postmenopausal women. Women in the intervention group, who received intensive counseling about their eating habits, cut their fat intake by an average of 18 grams a day during the five-year study, while the control group stayed at the same fat intake level. As you might expect, the intervention group also lost a bit of weight—about 6 pounds, on average. Those women lowered their risk of breast cancer recurrence by nearly 25%.

Longevity

Because excess weight plays a role in so many common and deadly diseases, being overweight and obese can cut years off your life. A study of more than one million adults showed that the lowest death rates were among people whose body mass indexes (BMIs) fell in the normal range (between 18.5 and 24.9; see Chapter 4). Having a BMI higher than 30, in contrast, can increase your risk of premature death two to three-fold. The degree of increased risk among overweight people has been questioned, but recent data gleaned from more than 527,000 adults between the ages of 50 and 71 found that being overweight at midlife raises the risk of premature death by 20% to 40%.

Answers to Test Your Knowledge Questions:

1. d
2. a
3. c
4. c

FOUR

Getting Ready:
Tools and Guidelines

If Americans were to make the effort to manage their weight using a variety of options, including better nutrition, more exercise, approved medications or even surgical approaches, we would be rewarded with significantly better health.

—Louis Aronne, M.D.,
director of the Comprehensive Weight-Control
Program and clinical associate professor
at the Weill Cornell Medical College

To start reaching your 10% goal, spend a bit of time getting mentally prepared, which really just means taking stock of the past and looking toward the future. Think about the reasons you've gained weight, as well as the reasons you want to lose weight. Consider not just the why, but also the where, when, and how. This chapter details a few key tools and habits you'll need to acquire and teaches you how to set realistic weight-loss goals. You'll also learn about partnering with health care professionals who can facilitate your journey.

IS YOUR HEAD IN THE GAME?

Start by taking an inventory of habits that might be contributing to your weight problem. Browse through the following lifestyle questions and consider the reasons for your answers. For example, if you answer yes to the first question in the "Eating" section, is it because you feel you're too busy to cook at home? The goal of this exercise isn't to tally up a score but rather to help you zero in on the areas that are most relevant for you. It will also introduce the crucial role of time management and sleep—two often-neglected aspects of weight loss.

Eating

If you answer yes to many of the following questions, you may be eating too much, eating too quickly, eating unhealthful foods, and have a tendency toward mindless and/or emotional eating. The solutions detailed in Chapters 5, 6, and 9 address these areas.

1. Do you eat out often?
2. Do you often eat fast food?
3. Do you ever feel stuffed or experience indigestion after meals?
4. Do you snack or eat a lot after dinner or late at night?
5. Do you eat when you are not hungry?
6. Do you drink regular soda, flavored coffee drinks, sports drinks, juices, sweetened packaged drinks, milkshakes, and smoothies once a day or more?
7. Do you often eat fried foods and processed foods (snacks and meats) more than just once in a while?
8. Do you often eat baked goods, pastries, bagels, and snacks like cookies, cake, and candy?
9. Does your home/school/office environment provide too many opportunities to eat unhealthfully?
10. Do you eat any main meals or snacks in front of the TV?
11. Do you eat while standing up?
12. Do you eat in front of your computer?
13. Do you eat to make yourself feel better emotionally?
14. Do you have trigger foods that cause you to overeat? If so, how often do you eat these foods?

Exercise

If you answer no to most of the following questions, you probably aren't getting enough physical activity. The solutions in Chapter 7 can get you moving.

1. Are you physically active at least thirty minutes a day most days of the week?
2. Do you enjoy physical activity, and if not, have you tried different types?
3. Do you ever wear a pedometer?
4. Do you go for walks?
5. Do you look for recreational/leisure activities that involve physical activity?
6. Do you feel you have time, motivation, and energy to exercise?
7. Do you walk or exercise with a partner?

Sleep

If you answer yes to most of the following questions, you may not be getting sufficient sleep, which can hamper weight loss. See Chapter 8 for advice in this area.

1. Do you sleep less than seven hours per night?
2. Do you usually go to bed and wake up at different times each day?
3. Do you eat heavy meals or snacks close to bedtime?
4. Do you watch TV right before bedtime?
5. Do you drink caffeinated beverages within six hours of bedtime?
6. Do you frequently drink alcohol before bedtime?

(continued)

7. Do you use your bed for activities other than sleep and sex?
8. Do you often wake up during the night?
9. Do you ever have trouble breathing during sleep time?
10. Do you have to take over-the-counter or prescription medications to help you fall asleep?
11. Do you feel fatigued throughout the day?
12. Do you think your level of tiredness negatively affects your eating or exercise habits?

Time Management, Lifestyle, and Stress

If you answer no to many of the first twelve questions and yes to the last two, you could likely benefit from better time management and stress management skills. Chapters 8 and 9 cover those topics.

1. Do you have time to prepare meals at home?
2. Do you have time to exercise?
3. Are eating well and exercising priorities in your life?
4. Do you pack snacks and lunches ahead of time?
5. Do you pack a gym bag the night before?
6. Do you go to the grocery store at least once a week?
7. Do you plan recreational activities on the weekends?
8. Do you spend time planning ahead for the next day or the whole week?
9. Do you have good time management habits?
10. Do you have a regular work schedule?
11. Do you avoid eating in your car or on your commute?
12. Do you bring your own food on the plane or when traveling?
13. Do you feel overwhelmed or very stressed?
14. Do your time constraints contribute to your stress level?

Another tool I give my patients is a chart that helps them take stock of their current habits and shows how unhealthful habits affect their daily life. Chances are many are familiar to you. Take a few minutes to look over the old habits, and think about whether the cost of changing them is worth the benefits you'll gain. What is most important to you: feeling less tired, looking better, or being stronger? If it's not already obvious, you'll soon realize that the benefits are all interconnected and tend to build upon one another.

	Old Habits		New Habits	
	Action	Effect	Cost to Fix the Problem	Benefit
Eating	Skipping breakfast	Midmorning energy slump and hunger, prone to snack on unhealthful breakfast treats	Eating cereal or toast for breakfast	Better appetite control, more energy
	Snacking on pastries and candy at work	Unhealthy weight, uncontrolled appetite, sugar crashes in the afternoon	Bring fresh and healthful prepacked snacks from home, avoid the office kitchen, go to bed earlier to avoid needing a caffeine or sugar boost in the afternoon	Healthier weight, boost in well-being and self-esteem
Exercising	Making excuses to avoid daily walks and exercise	Not reaping the benefits of more frequent exercise, gaining weight, feeling cranky and stressed	Exercising three or four times per week, packing a gym bag or placing sneakers near the door the night before	Improved energy, fitness, strength

(continued)

	Old Habits		New Habits	
	Action	**Effect**	**Cost to Fix the Problem**	**Benefit**
Sleeping	Sleeping only six hours per night	Daytime sleepiness, lack of energy, more prone to illnesses (colds, flu)	Go to bed earlier (watch less late-night television)	Feel more rested and energetic, less likely to get sick (infectious and chronic illnesses)
Time Management	Eating meals on the go	Feeling guilty and unhealthy after eating fast food or candy	Buy precut vegetables at the grocery store, give up some evening TV time to prepare and pack healthful lunches for next day	Healthier weight, boost in well-being and self-esteem

FROM TOOLBOX TO TARGET: THE FIRST FIVE STEPS

Now you're ready to crunch some numbers, with the help of a few tools and charts. In this section, you'll learn how to:

- Assemble your tools

- Chart your weight history

- Determine your set point and find your silhouette

- Identify your set point goal and calculate your target body weight

---

Set Point Toolbox

1. Accurate scale
2. Journal, ideally with a calendar
3. Timepiece (watch, stopwatch, or clock)
4. Comfortable walking shoes
5. Pedometer (optional)

Take 5 to Get 10

You probably already have the tools you need to get started. Here's more information on why you need them and how to use them:

1. An accurate scale. Weighing yourself daily takes very little effort and is perhaps the single most important thing you can do to reach and maintain a healthy weight. As I've said before, it's impossible to know exactly how many calories you eat and burn each day. That's why keeping tabs on your weight is the best way to know if your weight-loss efforts are working. Most people who lose weight say they weigh themselves frequently, often daily, according to the National Weight Control Registry, a self-selected database of people who have successfully lost weight. Several studies confirm this trend, including a 2006 study showing that people who weighed themselves daily regained about half as much weight as people who didn't weigh themselves every day. If you weigh yourself as part of your regular routine, you'll notice any weight gain and be able to take early action, rather than getting a wake-up call after you've gained 5 or 10 pounds.

I recommend a digital scale, because it's easy to read and can show even small weight changes. Some people like using specialized body fat monitor scales, which are more expensive but can provide extra motivation. Try weighing yourself every day, following these suggestions:

- Make sure your scale is on a flat, uncarpeted surface. Use the same scale every day to be consistent, because different scales (like the one at your doctor's office) may give a slightly different reading.

- Check that the scale's readings are consistent, giving the same weight when you step on, then off and on again.

- Weigh yourself at the same time of day, ideally in the morning after using the bathroom.

- Record your weight each day. Your food and activity log (see next tool) is a good place to write it down.

What's My Body Fat Percentage?

Some health clubs and doctors' offices have special scales that can calculate your body fat percentage. They exploit the fact that lean body mass conducts electricity faster than fat body mass, a concept known as bioelectric impedance. The scales use a small, harmless electrical current to measure the electrical resistance of the body, which is then used to calculate your body fat based on your height and weight. Body fat scales tend to be less accurate in people with obesity than in people who are slightly overweight or at a normal weight. Healthy adult men have body fat percentages between 10% and 25%, whereas the range for women is between 18% and 32%.

---

2. A journal to record your weight and keep a food and activity record. Writing down what you eat every day makes you more aware of the amount and type of foods you're eating and when you're eating them. This type of journaling has been proven to produce better and longer-lasting weight loss. Although some people enjoy this detail-oriented chore, others find it tedious, which is why I've developed a more streamlined technique: the R-K-O method. However, a more detailed food record can be helpful when you first start, as it can help you recognize situations or feelings that cause you to overindulge and learn to combat them. Common examples are environmental triggers (a fast-food restaurant or platter of donuts at the office) and emotional triggers (eating when you're tired, bored, or depressed).

The R-K-O Method

If you don't like recording every food item you eat, the R-K-O method works well. Most of my patients use it. At the beginning of every day, take stock of your eating and exercise efforts from the previous day by stepping on the scale.

- **R:** Each day that you follow a healthful diet and get enough physical activity is an R day of "regular reducing." You should see the effects of this on the scale, which should remain the same or go down, particularly if you have several R days in a row.
- **K:** What if you manage to keep your eating in check but don't get any exercise? That counts as a K day for "keeping it off." The same goes for when you exercise enough but eat more than you planned. Your weight will likely stay the same.
- **O:** Days when you splurge (particularly during holiday season) are O days for "off." The number on the scale will go up because you ate too much and/or didn't get enough physical activity.

The winning formula is a one-month review showing that R days outnumber K days and K days outnumber O days. To gauge the quality of the day based on your personal parameters, keep a general tally of your meals and serving sizes, which is explained Chapters 5 and 6. Similarly, a pedometer can help you keep track of your activity levels, as described in Chapter 7. The calendar is a sample of one of my patient's R-K-O journals. Mark was striving for 10,000 steps per day to meet his activity goals.

SAMPLE RKO CALENDAR FOR MARK
DECEMBER

Sunday	Monday	Tuesday	Wednesday	Thursday	Friday	Saturday
1	2	3	4	5	6	7
235 pounds	235 pounds	235 pounds	234 pounds	234 pounds	234 pounds	235 pounds
10,000 steps	8,000 steps	10,000 steps	10,000 steps	6,000 steps	4,000 steps	8,000 steps
Ate less	Ate less	On the road, ate more	Ate less	Ate less	Holiday party, ate more	Ate less
R	K	K	R	R	O	K
8	9	10	11	12	13	14
234 pounds	234 pounds	233 pounds				
10,000 steps	11,000 steps					
Ate less	Ate less					
R	_?_					

Pretend you're Mark. It's the morning of December 10, and you've just weighed yourself: 233 pounds. Looking back at yesterday's entry, would you give yourself an R, K, or O on December 9? The Appendix includes a blank R-K-O chart you can use for tracking your own progress.

3. A watch or clock. Paying attention to how much time you spend on specific activities throughout the day can help you manage your time more efficiently (see Chapter 8). A timepiece is also crucial for keeping track of progress toward your exercise goals.

4. Comfortable walking shoes. Walking is a simple, basic exercise almost everyone can do. You don't need to spend a lot of money; just choose shoes that offer comfort and support. If you have health issues or other physical limitations that make it difficult for you to walk more than short distances, see Chapter 7 for other options.

5. A pedometer or step counter (optional). This small, inexpensive device can be clipped onto a belt or clothing at your waist and will tell you how many steps you take in a day. You can estimate how far you travel as well, knowing that there are approximately 2,000 steps in 1 mile. You can use the information to track and gradually boost your activity level. In Chapter 7, you'll learn more about this and other ways to incorporate exercise into your daily life.

Your Weight History

To set your weight-loss goals, the first step is recognizing your own patterns of weight loss and gain, because it reveals your set point. Take a look at this sample weight history chart from Mark, who is 5'9" and 58 years old.

Current Weight	Highest Adult Weight	Lowest Adult Weight and Age	Weight at Age 21	Target Weight (10% loss)	Long-term Goal Weight and %
232 lb.	232 lb.	168 lb. age 28	195 lb.	209 lb. 23 lb. loss, 10% loss	200 lb. 32 lb. loss, 14% loss

As you can see from Mark's example, he lost weight but couldn't keep it off. Within 10 years, he had regained all of it. Mark set a long-term weight-loss goal of 32 pounds, or a 14% loss. A more reasonable target weight for him would be to lose 20 pounds and to hold steady at that weight for six months. After that, he can repeat the cycle once more until he reaches his 200-pound goal.

The best news is that a loss of 20 pounds is still enough to correct his weight-related health problems, which include high blood pressure and joint pain. Like Mark, you may also hope to eventually lose more than 10% of your current weight, perhaps down to what you weighed in your 20s. But there's no firm need to set a long-term goal unless you want to. For now, just focus on 10%.

Now, fill in your own weight history:

MY WEIGHT HISTORY CHART

Current Weight	Highest Adult Weight	Lowest Adult Weight and Age	Weight at Age 21	Target Weight (10% loss)

What's My Silhouette?

Now you're going to identify your body silhouette, which will give you a visual cue of your current and target set points. You probably know your blood pressure and cholesterol values; if not, schedule a physical with your primary care provider to get them. Your BMI number is an equally important vital sign, and determining your BMI is the first step to identifying your silhouette.

Step 1. Determine your BMI

Body mass index (BMI) is a measure of body size based on height and weight that applies to adult men and women. Health care providers use this standard tool to determine whether a person is a normal weight, overweight (equal to about 20–40 pounds of excess fat), or obese (equal to about 40–100 or more pounds of excess fat). These categories are based on several studies involving millions of people to correlate BMI values with rates of illness and death. The healthiest values—that is, the values with the lowest rates of illness and death—are between 19 and 25 for men and between 18 and 25 for women. That's why people with BMIs in this healthiest range are considered to be of "normal" weight.

But be aware that BMI values don't tell the whole story. One problem with using BMI is that very muscular people may fall into the overweight category when they are actually healthy and fit. Another is that people who have lost muscle mass, such as older people, may be in the healthy weight category when they may actually fall short in terms of their nutrient reserves and fitness. So while BMI is useful as a general measurement of size and for tracking trends in the population, it's not a good way to determine an individual's health status. For that, you need to know not only your body size but also the quality of your diet, your fitness level, and any health risks you may have.

The simplest way to find your BMI is to look it up in the table. Or use a Web-based calculator at http://nhlbisupport.com/bmi/. If you're curious about the formula, you can calculate your BMI yourself:

1. Measure your height in inches (without shoes) and your weight in pounds (without clothing).

2. Multiply your weight by 703.

3. Divide that number by your height.

4. Divide again by your height.

Once you've determined your BMI, circle the number on the table.

BODY MASS INDEX														
BMI	**19**	**20**	**21**	**22**	**23**	**24**	**25**	**26**	**27**	**28**	**29**	**30**	**35**	**40**
Height	**Weight in Pounds**													
4'10"	91	96	100	105	110	115	119	124	129	134	138	143	167	191
4'11"	94	99	104	109	114	119	124	128	133	138	143	148	173	198
5'0"	97	102	107	112	118	123	128	133	138	143	148	153	179	204
5'1"	100	106	111	116	122	127	132	137	143	148	153	158	185	211
5'2"	104	109	115	120	126	131	136	142	147	153	158	164	191	218
5'3"	107	113	118	124	130	135	141	146	152	158	163	169	197	225
5'4"	110	116	122	128	134	140	145	151	157	163	169	174	204	232
5'5"	114	120	126	132	138	144	150	156	162	168	174	180	210	240
5'6"	118	124	130	136	142	148	155	161	167	173	179	186	216	247
5'7"	121	127	134	140	146	153	159	166	172	178	185	191	223	255
5'8"	125	131	138	144	151	158	164	171	177	184	190	197	230	262
5'9"	128	135	142	149	155	162	169	176	182	189	196	203	236	270
5'10"	132	139	146	153	160	167	174	181	188	195	202	207	243	278
5'11"	136	143	150	157	165	172	179	186	193	200	208	215	250	286
6'0"	140	147	154	162	169	177	184	191	199	206	213	221	258	294
6'1"	144	151	159	166	174	182	189	197	204	212	219	227	265	302
6'2"	148	155	163	171	179	186	194	202	210	218	225	233	272	311
6'3"	152	160	168	176	184	192	200	208	216	224	232	240	279	319
6'4"	156	164	172	180	189	197	205	213	221	230	238	246	287	328

NOTE: The Appendix has a chart that includes BMIs between 41 and 54. If your BMI is higher than 40, see a doctor who specializes in treating severe obesity before using this book.

Step 2. Identify your silhouette number

Using your BMI, locate your present silhouette number from the silhouette charts on pages 68 through 71.

Step 3. Identify your target silhouette

This is one step below your current silhouette.

Step 4. Find your target body weight

1. Multiply current body weight by 0.1 (160 lb. × 0.1 = 16 lb.).

2. Subtract that value from current weight (160 − 16 = 144 lb.).

3. The answer is your target body weight (144 lb.), and the 10% (16 lb.) is your target six-month weight-loss goal. Fill this in on your weight history chart.

Step 5. Spend at least six months reaching and maintaining your new target set point

Use the plans and advice outlined in the rest of the book to attain your goal body weight, losing no more than a pound or two per week.

Step 6. Don't give up your 10% for anything!

That is, don't change a thing! Some people are so excited by their initial 10% weight loss that they get a little greedy and either go back to their bad habits or try to lose more weight too quickly. Once you've arrived at your goal set point, just keep doing what you are doing. This will help you hold your weight at its new set point, which is crucial before trying to lose more weight. For some people, maintaining new, healthful life-style habits will actually help them move down to the next set point.

Step 7. Repeat the previous steps to lose additional weight, if desired

When you've maintained your target weight for six months, copy the weight history chart. Fill it in with your new, lower target weight.

FEMALE VERTICAL SILHOUETTES

Silhouette	Silhouette Number	BMI	Sample Weight for 5'4" Woman
	1	18 19 20	110 lb. +/−3 lb.
	2	21 22 23	128 lb. +/−3 lb.
	3	24 25 26	145 lb. +/−3 lb.
	4	27 28 29	163 lb. +/−3 lb.
	5	30 31 32	180 lb. +/−3 lb.

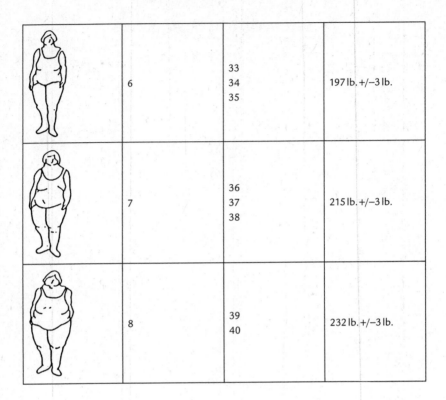

	6	33 34 35	197 lb. +/−3 lb.
	7	36 37 38	215 lb. +/−3 lb.
	8	39 40	232 lb. +/−3 lb.

MALE VERTICAL SILHOUETTES

Silhouette	Set Point Number	BMI	Sample Weight for 5'9" Man
	1	18 19 20	128 lb. +/−3 lb.
	2	21 22 23	149 lb. +/−3 lb.
	3	24 25 26	169 lb. +/−3 lb.
	4	27 28 29	189 lb. +/−3 lb.
	5	30 31 32	209 lb. +/−3 lb.

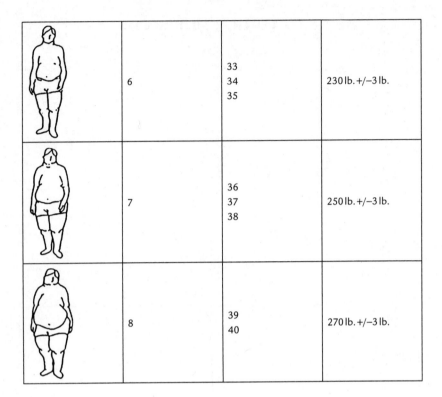

	6	33 34 35	230 lb. +/−3 lb.
	7	36 37 38	250 lb. +/−3 lb.
	8	39 40	270 lb. +/−3 lb.

WORKING WITH HEALTH CARE PROVIDERS

Given the many health concerns related to excess weight, it makes sense to work with your primary care provider (PCP), which may be a doctor, nurse practitioner, or physician's assistant. People are often hesitant to discuss weight issues with their PCPs and vice versa. Some PCPs avoid the topic for fear of insulting their patients while others simply believe they have nothing to offer in terms of advice. Finding a supportive PCP can make a world of difference. I realize that people sometimes have limited choices when it comes to selecting a PCP due to availability, insurance, or other issues. If you're fortunate to have one you like, that's great. If you're in the

market for a new one, here are two questions you should ask him or her:

1. Do you have experience monitoring and counseling people who are trying to lose weight?

2. Can you refer me to other specialists who can assist me with weight loss, such as dietitians and behavioral therapists? (See "Allied Health Care Professionals" later in this chapter.)

Patient-Oriented Treatment

Fortunately, many PCPs are changing the way they talk to their patients in an effort to make patients feel more comfortable and improve communication. Ultimately, having a good rapport with your doctor depends on many things. Clinicians trained in patient-oriented weight management learn specific skills and qualities. For example, they should:

- Start a conversation about nutrition status or weight loss by first asking your permission

- Actively listen to your medical history and concerns without interruption

- Use language and terms that are clear to you

- Repeat their messages several times and in a variety of ways

- Provide a clear action plan with specifics on the timing of follow-up visits, calls, or emails

- Allow sufficient time to answer your questions

Patient-centered counseling encourages patients to set goals and express their own ideas for therapy, with input from their health care provider. The plan you devise with your provider should include realistic goals that take your personal situation into account. Ideally, you should have follow-up visits or some sort of contact at least four times a year so that your PCP can monitor your progress, modify the treatment plan if needed, and provide encouragement.

Motivational Interviewing

A related skill that's become more widespread is motivational interviewing (MI). Clinicians trained in MI adopt a nonjudgmental, encouraging approach that allows you to discuss the positive and negative aspects of your behavior. MI is similar to but less formal than traditional talk therapy, in which you meet regularly with a therapist to discuss your problems. (Chapter 9 includes more detailed information about therapy and counseling for weight loss.) A skilled practitioner of MI allows you to do most of the talking and shows respect, support, and encouragement as you describe your challenges and motivations to change (or not to change). The success of MI lies partly with the skill of the clinician but also in your willingness to talk.

Do your best to be open and forthcoming about your weight issues. You can take the initiative by starting the conversation. For example, you could tell your PCP that you'd like some help figuring our how to reach a healthy weight and ask for suggestions and advice. Or you might mention that you've heard that BMI can determine your health status and that you'd like to discuss your own weight and BMI value.

Making the Most of Your Visit

Your yearly checkup is an ideal time to talk with your PCP about a weight-loss plan. In addition to a standard physical exam, your PCP should order standard age-appropriate screening tests, such as blood pressure, cholesterol, Pap test, mammogram, and forth. Your medical history should include questions about the health of your first-degree relatives (parents and siblings). Be sure to mention if anyone in your family has a history of overweight or weight-related diseases, such as type 2 diabetes or high blood pressure.

Because a doctor's visit is usually quite short, make the most of your time together by coming prepared. Be sure to bring:

1. Your weight history chart. It may offer clues as to the causes—and best solutions—for your weight problem. Note any major weight losses and gains and diets you have tried.

2. A list of all the medications you're currently taking, including prescription and over-the-counter drugs, as well as vitamins and other dietary supplements. Be sure to note the frequency and dosage of each product. If you have more than a few, it may be simpler to bring the bottles with you to your appointment.

A new trend among doctors is to use a prescription pad to write down simple advice about diet and exercise, which you can post some-place you'll see it often, like the refrigerator door. You can talk with your PCP about mixed feelings you may have about making lifestyle changes to lose weight. For example, your spouse or family might be resistant to dietary changes and might insist on keeping junk food in the house. Or perhaps you don't enjoy exercising and worry that you won't be able to find an exercise routine you can sustain.

Allied Health Care Professionals

The most successful treatments for many chronic health conditions often involve a team of specialists. The same is true for excess weight. Allied health care professionals, which include nurses, medical assistants, die-titians, psychologists, social workers, and physical therapists, can help you address specific issues about diet, behavior, and exercise. Dietitians can help you create and follow a healthy eating plan that will enable you to lose weight. If physical problems due to a medical condition or injury make physical activity challenging, a physical therapist can help. And cognitive behavioral therapists can address emotional or behavioral is-sues that may be hindering your weight-loss attempts. (More details on these professionals are featured in Chapters 6 through 9.) Your insurance plan will dictate how many visits are covered per year. Don't be shy about seeking help from allied health care professionals. In many cases, they are less expensive and more available than PCPs. Finding the right combination of medical support and therapy can make it easier (and more enjoyable) to stick to your weight-loss plan.

Group Appointments: An Innovative Approach

Yet another new trend in health care consists of a group office visit, which can increase the amount of time you interact with your doctor. Two common examples are cooperative health care clinics (CHCC) and drop-in group medical appointments (DIGMA). With this approach, six to eight patients receive consecutively, staggered appointments at the end of the day—for example, from 4:00 P.M. to 5:30 P.M. When you arrive, nurses or medical assistants measure your vital signs and discuss your main problems privately with you. You then go to an exam room where the clinician conducts an interactive group assessment, during which you can discuss your shared, nonprivate problems. Each person has a chance to speak to the clinician privately for five to eight minutes while another facilitator continues the group session. You receive a total of ninety minutes of individual and group interaction with your doctor.

Physicians often find this model makes it easier to manage their large patient loads, and patients report that they receive more information and support than they would have during a brief office visit. It's a good approach for people who find support in numbers and can be particularly helpful in the context of treating weight-related issues. You may want to find a doctor's office that uses this approach or suggest it to your own doctor.

Weight-loss Medications and Surgery

The National Institutes of Health (NIH) has set guidelines for the appropriate use of weight-loss interventions. Weight-loss medications should only be taken by people who have a BMI of 30 or higher, or in the case of those with weight-related health problems, a BMI of 27 or more, as detailed in the table. For people with BMIs lower than 27, the risks of these medications likely outweigh the benefits. It's worth noting that these medications don't necessarily work for everyone. People who don't lose at least a pound a week in the first month on a weight-loss medication probably won't be helped by the drug. Note, too, that regardless of your BMI, diet, physical activity, and behavior therapy are the cornerstone treatments. You can't achieve lasting weight loss with a drug or an operation alone, because neither will work if you don't change the way you eat, exercise, and behave for the rest of your life. The Appendix includes additional information about weight-loss medications and surgeries.

A GUIDE TO SELECTING TREATMENT

	BMI Category				
Treatment	**25–26.9**	**27–29.9**	**30–34.9**	**35–39.9**	**≥40**
Diet, physical activity, and behavior therapy	With related diseases or conditions*		+		
Drug treatment		With related diseases or conditions*	+		
Surgery			With related diseases or conditions*		

Source: Modified from *The Practical Guide: Identification, Evaluation, and Treatment of Overweight and Obesity in Adults* (NHLBI and NAASO). NIH Publication Number 00484, October 2000.

*Related diseases (often called comorbidities) include heart disease, type 2 diabetes, and sleep apnea. The *conditions* refer to other factors that put you at risk for these diseases (known as risk factors), such as cigarette smoking, high blood pressure, elevated LDL ("bad") cholesterol, low HDL ("good") cholesterol, elevated blood sugar level, or an increased waist circumference (35 inches or higher for women, 40 inches or higher for men). People with two or more of these conditions qualify. Doctors usually prescribe drug treatment only if you have not lost 1 pound per week after six months of diet, physical activity, and behavioral therapy.

⁺Use of indicated treatment regardless of related diseases or conditions.

FIVE

Eat Less and Shed Pounds

More Americans are fatter than ever, and one thing contributing to the problem is "portion distortion." Research studies now show that portion size affects energy intake—the larger the portion, the more calories people are likely to eat at any one time.

—Karen Donato, M.S., R.D.,
coordinator of the National Health Obesity Education
Initiative for the National Heart,
Lung, and Blood Institute (NHLBI)

MARY'S STORY: EATING LESS, ONE SMALL STEP AT A TIME

Mary came to our nutrition medicine clinic in mid-January, seeking help with her New Year's resolution to trim her expanding waistline. She'd gained several pounds over the holidays. The year had been especially bad—in fact, she'd gained nearly 15 pounds since September and could no longer fit into many of her clothes. Eating too many sweets and other high-calorie goodies at holiday parties was part of the problem. But my conversation with her revealed another key piece of information: Mary's twin boys (her only children) had left for college in September.

Mary and her husband had empty nest syndrome and showed some of the classic symptoms: grocery shopping, preparing food, and eating as if there were still four people in the house. Mary had gone overboard when her boys came home for the holidays, celebrating with three weeks of feasts and treats. When they returned to school in January, Mary turned to food for comfort. This emotional eating is another common reason people struggle with weight gain.

Mary, who is 5'3", had weighed 125 pounds before having the twins when she was 29. By the time they left for college, she had gained 20 pounds—slightly more than 1 pound per year, which is average for American adults. Adding the 15 pounds she'd put on in the past few months, she was tipping the scales at 160 pounds at age 47.

Mary needed a complete diet makeover. The first step was encouraging her to adapt her shopping and cooking habits. Because her boys had been athletic in high school, she often prepared heavy, filling meals, like lasagna and chili. We suggested that she use less meat and cheese and instead include more vegetables in her recipes to make lighter versions of these favorite dishes (see the Appendix for more examples). She also started preparing new, less filling meals such as fish, which she and her husband both enjoyed. When they went out to dinner, they tried Chinese and Thai restaurants, choosing dishes that were heavy on the vegetables with small amounts of meat. And Mary gave up her habit of baking cookies and brownies, except for special occasions when guests could share the treats.

She was more careful to control the amount of food she prepared. If she made more than she and her husband could eat in one meal, she would immediately freeze the leftovers for another meal. To cut down on how much they ate at each meal, Mary and her husband started using smaller plates.

During this first month, we contacted Mary by email to discuss food exchanges, monitor meal planning, and offer encouragement. By her second clinic visit, she had mastered enough new eating habits to prevent further weight gain. Now, she was ready to start losing. To maintain her weight of 160 pounds, I calculated that Mary was eating about 2,400 calories a day (160 lb. × 15 calories/lb. = 2,400 calories). As with all of my patients, I advised an easy-does-it approach, suggesting tips for making small, gradual changes that she could keep up for the rest of her life.

I recommended that Mary cut out approximately one-eighth of her daily food intake, which is approximately 10% of her calories. For

Mary, that translated to about 240 calories, or the amount in one candy bar. We agreed that measuring and recording her weight every morning would be a good way to monitor her progress and that it would be easy to communicate via email.

Mary used a variety of new techniques to eat less. To leave one-eighth of each meal behind, she put a few forkfuls of food onto a separate salad plate before she started eating, which she would either save for another meal or throw away. She liked this strategy because she could still eat her favorite foods and she didn't feel deprived. And by also incorporating slow eating (one of my two mealtime rules), she soon found that she really didn't miss the small extra amount.

Second, she changed her snacking habits. Every afternoon, Mary ate a brownie or a baked good with a cup of tea, a habit left over from when she baked treats for her boys to eat after school. She wasn't necessarily hungry when she ate these treats, but she had grown used to having a daily sweet. Knowing that these items contain at least 200 calories each, Mary acknowledged that by cutting them out, she would save 10% of her calories right there. But she didn't want to completely abandon this familiar ritual—and she didn't have to. On days when she didn't feel like reducing the portions at each meal, she would skip her afternoon treat. Other days when she craved an afternoon snack, she would cut back in some other way. Somewhere along the way, Mary realized she could substitute the baked good with a lower-calorie, healthier option, like a piece of fruit or a cup of low-fat yogurt.

Mary was also a late-night snacker. In the previous months, she had spent the evenings snacking her way through leftovers from dinner (that is, what would have been her boys' dinner portions). In years past, she indulged in homework snacks that she bought for her sons, like popcorn and ice cream. She started buying gum instead of the snacks, because she found that chewing gum after dinner was a great way to keep food out of her mouth. When the gum trick became stale, she realized that brushing her teeth had the same effect. She also encouraged her husband to distract her from sneaking into the kitchen.

Together, these tricks helped her cut way back on her late-night, high-fat snacking habit.

Finally, Mary tried to keep track of her eating routines by keeping a simple food journal. But she didn't like listing all of the foods she ate every day, so I introduced her to my R-K-O method (see Chapter 4). With these tools in hand, bolstered by emails and personal doctor's visits, Mary was able to move toward her goal of losing 16 pounds (10% of her body weight). Within three months, by the end of May, she had lost 8 pounds—just in time to enjoy her family all together again for the summer. Feeling and looking better gave her the motivation to ramp up her efforts over the summer, and she easily met her six-month goal without the relapses she'd experienced in her earlier attempts.

EATING LESS: THE FIRST STEP

There's no getting around it: to lose weight, you've got to eat less. All weight-loss programs limit calories one way or another. Even the once-popular, low-carbohydrate Atkins diet limited calories by almost completely eliminating a major food group. Average Americans get 50% to 55% percent of their calories from carbohydrates. Some carbohydrates, such as whole-grain bread, brown rice, baked potatoes, and carrots, are packed with healthful nutrients. But many of the most popular carb-rich foods—white bread, french fries, cookies, donuts, and candy—tend to be quite high in fat and calories and low in nutrients.

By completely avoiding carbohydrates, a person will often eat far fewer calories (up to 1,000 fewer a day) and will therefore lose weight quickly. The trouble is, you can't stick to that regimen for very long, which is one reason a lot of people who initially lose weight on a low-carb diet end up regaining it. What's more, completely eliminating a major food group from your diet will leave you deprived, bored, and vulnerable to food cravings and hunger. You'll miss out on key nutrients and the enjoyment of eating a well-rounded diet. You don't have to completely give up pizza or candy or other foods you love. Like Mary, you just have to learn ways to eat fewer calories overall.

To set yourself up for success, I recommend that you focus only on eating less for the time being. Don't worry about what foods you're eating or how much physical activity you're getting. We'll get to that soon enough. Any time you learn a new skill, it's much easier and more effective to break it down into smaller, more manageable pieces. The great news is that the skills you learn in Chapter 6, about choosing healthful foods, as well as Chapter 7, the exercise chapter, will make it even easier for you to eat less, because healthful foods fill you up and exercise curbs your appetite.

Remember, there's no rush: the more you can embrace the easy-does-it approach, the more likely you'll be to succeed over the long term. It took years to gain the weight, and it will take time to get to your target weight. Take at least one month to practice the new skills detailed in this chapter and see if you can start racking up R days in your journal. Later, we'll expand the definition of an R day to include healthy foods and activity. But for now, just consider eating less as your weight-loss aspect of the plan when rating your day.

Two Rules for Eating Less

As any veteran dieter knows, eating less can leave you hungry, but usually only if you drastically reduce how much you're eating. Remember, you've got to work with your set point, not against it. If you get too hungry, you're more likely to scarf down whatever's within closest reach, which may be a giant muffin on the conference table at work or a leftover cupcake in the fridge. But hunger isn't the only problem. The siren song of a sweet treat (or a plate of french fries, if that's more your style) can tempt you even when you're not hungry. Fortunately, two strategies can help you avoid both of these pitfalls.

Which Diet Is Best? The One That Works for You

Researchers who've compared different diets in head-to-head studies have found that it's not the specific diet plan you choose but whether you stick with it that makes the difference. For example, one study compared four popular diets: the Atkins diet (a low-carbohydrate diet); the Ornish diet (a very-low fat, mainly vegetarian diet); Weight Watchers (a low-calorie diet that uses a point system); and the Zone diet (a diet based on specific combinations of protein, carbohydrate, and fat). Researchers randomly assigned 160 overweight or obese people to one of the diets. After one year, nearly half of the participants had dropped out of the study. But those who completed the study lost similar amounts of weight (about 5 to 7 pounds each, on average, no matter which diet they were on). People in the Atkins and Ornish groups were more likely to drop out of the study, probably because they found these plans too extreme. Note that for some people, the structure of a restricted plan may be helpful. But for others, it can backfire (see "Rigid Control" later in this chapter).

Other studies support the popular notion that a low-carb, high-protein diet leads to quicker weight loss than a low-fat diet. But in the studies that lasted for a year or longer, average weight loss was about the same regardless of diet type. And averages can mask some startling individual differences. In one trial of both low-carb and low-fat diets, some people lost weight while others gained. In the low-fat group, some people lost weight (one more than 50 pounds), while other people gained weight—up to 30 pounds, in one case! In the low-carb group, the individual differences ranged from 65 pounds lost to 18 pounds gained. These findings reinforce the idea that one size doesn't fit all when it comes to choosing a diet. What works well for your best friend may not be a great fit for you.

Rule 1. Feel full with 450

To feel full and satisfied until your next meal (usually about four hours later), you should eat at least 450 calories at each meal. The science behind the 450-calorie suggestion comes from a study in which women rated their feelings of hunger and fullness before and after eating a pasta dish that contained between 440 and 463 calories. The dishes featured different types of protein, including tofu or chicken, as well as tomatoes, cheese, olives, and artichoke hearts. Graphs of changes in the women's hunger levels suggest that while hunger levels gradually rise after eating, they don't reach premeal hunger levels until about four hours after eating.

HUNGER AFTER A MEAL

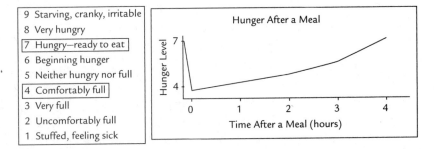

After eating a filling meal of at least 450 calories, people usually don't reach their premeal hunger levels for about four hours.

As you probably know from personal experience, if you eat a small morning meal (a cup of coffee and a piece of toast, for instance), you'll probably be hungry well before midday. Many people say they're not hungry in the morning. However, if you eat less at dinner and curb your evening and late-night snacking, you may find that you're hungrier when you wake up in the morning. Also, many studies show that eating breakfast can boost weight-loss (and weight maintenance) efforts. For breakfast and lunch menus that contain around 450 calories, see the recipes in the Appendix.

Keep in mind that 450 is the minimum number of calories you need at one meal. Most people eat the bulk of their daily calories—usually 700 to 800 calories or more—during their evening meal. Even if you ate 450 calories at breakfast, 600 at lunch, and 800 at dinner, your total for the day would be 1,850. That's less than what I recommended for Mary (2,400–240=2,160). She'd still have 310 calories left over for snacks.

As I've said before, I don't want you to get too hung up on keeping track of your calories. The Nutrition Facts panel on all packaged foods can give you an idea of the number of calories in many foods. But most of us eat a mix of fresh, homemade, and packaged foods, in addition to the prepared foods we buy in snack bars and restaurants, few of which provide calorie or other nutrition information on their food offerings. The jumbo-sized portions common in fast-food and other eating establishments make it even more difficult to guess the number of calories in a given meal or food item—even for trained dietitians!

Rule 2. Take 20

Another secret to eating less is to spend at least twenty minutes eating each meal. The gut hormones and stretch receptors in your stomach that send an "I'm full" message take fifteen to twenty minutes to reach your brain. Don't drown out these important messages by eating too quickly. If you can train yourself to eat slowly, you won't crave a second helping.

When volunteers in a study at the University of Rhode Island were asked to eat a large dish of pasta quickly, just until they reached a point of comfortable fullness, they gobbled down an average of 646 calories

Calorie Confusion

How many calories are in a 2-cup serving of lasagna? Let's see; it has noodles, tomato sauce, cheese, maybe some meat and vegetables. Even if you have a rough idea of how many calories are in each of those items and can estimate the amounts of each in a 2-cup serving, could you even come close to guessing the total calories? Probably not. Even trained professionals have a tough time estimating calories in restaurant entrees, according to a study that asked dietitians to guess the number of calories in several popular restaurant meals, such as a chicken Caesar salad, a 10-ounce hamburger and 11 onion rings, and an 11-ounce tuna salad sandwich. The dietitians low-balled the calories in every case—in one case by nearly 700 calories. For instance, they judged the hamburger and onion-ring meal to be 865 calories, when it was actually 1,550.

Another study found that people often underestimate calories in large fast-food meals. Trained interviewers asked patrons of a fast-food restaurant to estimate the calories in the meals they'd just eaten. The interviewers then calculated the actual calorie counts, by surreptitiously gathering up the empty cartons and wrappers from the patron's trays. In a second phase of the study, undergraduates were asked to guess the calories in various-sized combo meals of chicken nuggets, fries, and cola, which ranged from 445 to 1,780 calories for each meal. The customers and students proved quite accurate when guessing the calories in normal-sized meals, missing the mark by only 2% to 3%. But they underestimated the calories in larger meals by 23% to 38%. Although these trends were true for both normal and overweight people, overweight people were more likely to order larger meals and therefore tend to overeat more often.

What's the message here? You don't have to avoid fast-food restaurants. You can't estimate (or control) the calories in the food you order, but you can control your portion size. Order the smallest size—and just because you receive your food speedily doesn't mean you have to eat it quickly! Chapter 6 includes more information about making healthy choices at restaurants.

in about nine minutes. On another day, researchers served the same meal but asked the volunteers to eat slowly and to put down their forks between each bite. This time, the volunteers took an average of twenty-nine minutes during their unhurried meal and ate an average of 579 calories each. They also said they enjoyed the meal more when they ate it slowly.

Have you ever sat down to dinner and been interrupted midmeal by a phone call? If it wasn't a telemarketer but someone you actually wanted to speak with, chances are you weren't quite as hungry when you sat back down to your meal ten minutes later. Your gut hormones had already started working. Other tactics to help you eat more slowly

THE TWENTY-MINUTE PLATE

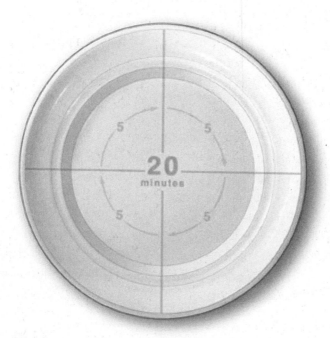

Visually divide your plate into four sections and give yourself five minutes to eat the first section. Begin on the second section only after those first five minutes are up. Repeat for the next two sections so that it takes twenty minutes to finish.

are chewing each mouthful well and talking with tablemates. I've also found that sipping a glass of wine during dinner is a pleasant way to help savor the meal in a more leisurely way.

Another great technique is to practice mindful eating, which means bringing a keen awareness and appreciation to what you are eating and why. Focus your attention on the present moment, which requires deliberate concentration. When you sit down to eat, take a moment to check in with your feelings. Are you truly hungry or is it just time to eat? Are you happy and calm or tense and anxious? Take time to relish each bite, noticing how your food looks, smells, tastes, and feels. Practicing mindful eating may help prevent mindless eating and emotional eating, as described in more detail in Chapter 9.

A stopwatch or kitchen timer comes in handy to train yourself to spend twenty minutes on a meal.

THE EATING INVENTORY: ARE YOU FLEXIBLE OR RIGID?

The challenge of eating less may not be so much about avoiding hunger. It may be about avoiding circumstances that tempt you to eat when you're not hungry. In addition to hunger, two other factors—disinhibition and dietary restraint—affect how much you eat. As I described in Chapter 2, disinhibition is a term researchers use to describe uncontrolled eating, which is also sometimes referred to as emotional eating. Stress, depression, anxiety, and drinking alcohol are common triggers for this loss of control. Dietary restraint refers to the practice of deliberately controlling how much you undereat. Together, these three factors (perceived hunger, disinhibition, and dietary restraint) make up the Eating Inventory (EI), a questionnaire developed in the mid-1980s.

Researchers use EI scores to identify both positive and negative behaviors linked to weight-loss efforts. For example, a higher dietary restraint score means you're more likely to be successful at losing and keeping off weight. A high disinhibition score, however, means you're more likely to abandon all restraint and overeat, and you're also more likely to have a hard time controlling your weight.

Back to Balance

When you begin to eat less, you'll be in dietary restraint mode. But as it turns out, there's a right and a wrong way to restrain yourself. A more detailed EI questionnaire, developed by German researchers, teased out these differences. If you control your eating very strictly—for example, you never allow yourself to have any of your favorite treats—you'll be more likely to fail at your weight-loss efforts. But if you practice a more flexible type of restrained eating, you're less likely to disinhibit and more likely to succeed at your weight-loss efforts.

To see whether you tend to be more rigid or flexible, first read both of the following questionnaires to the end without marking your answers. Notice the similarities between the two lists. Both focus solely on behaviors and perceptions about food and eating less. You'll also notice some subtle differences. Then go back and circle your answers on both questionnaires.

Flexible Control

1. When I have eaten my quota of calories, I am usually good about not eating any more. (<u>true</u>-false)

2. I deliberately take small helpings as a means of weight control. (<u>true</u>-false)

3. While on a diet, if I eat food that is not allowed, I consciously eat less for a period of time to make up for it. (<u>true</u>-false)

4. I consciously hold back at meals in order not to gain weight. (<u>true</u>-false)

5. I pay a great deal of attention to changes in my figure. (<u>true</u>-false)

6. How conscious are you of what you are eating? (not at all, <u>slightly, moderately, extremely</u>)

7. How likely are you to consciously eat less than you want? (unlikely, slightly likely, <u>moderately likely, very likely</u>)

8. If I eat a little bit more on one day, I make up for it the next day. (<u>true</u>-false)

9. I pay attention to my figure, but I still enjoy a variety of foods. (<u>true</u>-false)

10. I prefer light foods that are not fattening. (<u>true</u>-false)

11. If I eat a little bit more during one meal, I make up for it at the next meal. (<u>true</u>-false)

12. Do you deliberately restrict your intake during meals, even though you would like to eat more? (<u>always, often,</u> rarely, never)

Rigid Control

1. I have a pretty good idea of the number of calories in common foods. (<u>true</u>-false)

2. I count calories as a conscious means of controlling my weight. (<u>true</u>-false)

3. How often are you dieting in a conscious effort to control your weight? (rarely, sometimes, <u>usually, always</u>)

4. Would a weight fluctuation of 5 pounds affect the way you live your life? (not at all, slightly, <u>moderately, very much</u>)

5. Do feelings of guilt about overeating help you to control your food intake? (never, rarely, <u>often, always</u>)

6. How frequently do you avoid stocking up on tempting foods? (almost never, seldom, <u>usually, almost always</u>)

7. How likely are you to shop for low-calorie foods? (unlikely, slightly likely, <u>moderately likely, very likely</u>)

8. I eat diet foods, even if they do not taste very good. (<u>true</u>-false)

9. A diet would be too boring a way for me to lose weight. (<u>true</u>-false)

10. I would rather skip a meal than stop eating in the middle of one. (<u>true</u>-false)

11. I alternate between times when I diet strictly and times when I don't pay much attention to what and how much I eat. (<u>true</u>-false)

12. Sometimes I skip meals to avoid gaining weight. (<u>true</u>-false)

13. I avoid some foods on principle even though I like them. (<u>true</u>-false)

14. I try to stick to a plan when I lose weight. (<u>true</u>-false)

15. Without a diet plan, I wouldn't know how to control my weight. (<u>true</u>-false)

16. Quick success is most important for me during a diet. (<u>true</u>-false)

If you circled more of the underlined answers in the first questionnaire, you tend to have more flexible control, which is linked with a lower likelihood of disinhibition. If you circled more of the underlined answers in the second questionnaire, you tend to take a more rigid approach to weight loss and probably have a greater tendency to disinhibit. That's okay. This chapter and those that follow will help you learn to become more flexible with your eating habits.

CONQUERING DISINHIBITION

One way to avoid gorging on your favorite treats is to allow yourself to eat small amounts of these goodies on a regular basis. If you crave chocolate, enjoy a small square every day. Training yourself to stop after just a small amount can be tricky at first. But eventually, you may find that your cravings subside with this more flexible attitude.

See if you can begin to notice if certain things other than hunger trigger you to eat. Sometimes, people eat when they're actually thirsty rather than hungry. Emotional triggers—feeling bored, lonely, or frustrated—may set off an eating spree. The mere presence of tempting foods (pizza dripping with cheese, a frosted chocolate brownie, or any favorite food) will entice most people to indulge even if they don't feel the least bit hungry. As I've noted before, alcohol is another common cause of disinhibition. Drinking that second or third glass of wine during dinner makes you likely to abandon all restraint and overeat. Combine two or more of these circumstances and you'll be squarely on track for an O or "off" day. Don't beat yourself up if you end up with an O day in your journal once in while. But if this becomes a pattern, you need a strategy for change. The harsh reality is that just one extreme O day—eating an entire pint of ice cream, for instance—can cancel out a week's worth of hard-earned R days. If you find that you often eat excessive amounts of food, especially in response to emotional triggers, you may have binge eating disorder.

Chapter 9 addresses the emotional aspects of overeating in greater detail. It also explains some of the behavior-changing techniques used by the dietitians who coach the participants in our diet studies. For the time being, just try to be more aware of situations that cause you to disinhibit. Is it the all-you-can eat buffet at the Indian restaurant near your office? Or maybe it's the monthly potluck at your book group, where everyone brings an appetizer or dessert to share. Or perhaps you're like Mary, who sneaks into the kitchen after dinner to nibble on leftovers. If brushing your teeth or chewing gum doesn't do the trick, you might even try putting a physical barrier (a chair or a piece of masking tape, for example) in front of your kitchen door to remind yourself to stay out. Be flexible and creative, and remember that every little bit of effort helps. Making a number of small changes will translate into a noticeable weight loss.

Binge Eating: Out-of-Control Disinhibition

People who frequently gorge themselves—and feel out of control while doing so—may have binge eating disorder. Although not formally recognized as a mental disorder by the American Psychiatric Association, experts have proposed adding binge eating disorder to the *Diagnostic and Statistical Manual of Mental Disorders* (DSM-IV). A 2007 study reported that about one in thirty-five Americans have binge eating disorder, making it more common that other better-known eating disorders such as anorexia nervosa and bulimia.

Binge eating is more common among women and is strongly linked with obesity, although most people with obesity do not have binge eating disorder. Some characteristics of the disorder include eating quickly, often to the point of discomfort or pain; frequently eating alone; hoarding food and hiding empty food containers; and feeling depressed, disgusted, or upset about the amount eaten. Depression and anxiety are common among people with binge eating disorder. The proposed DSM-IV description for the disorder includes binge eating that occurs at least two days a week for six months.

Less than half of those with binge eating disorder seek treatment for the problem, and doctors typically don't ask their patients about possible bingeing habits. That's unfortunate, because psychotherapy, especially cognitive behavioral therapy or CBT (see Chapter 9), can help. If you think you might have binge eating disorder, ask your health care professional for a referral to a therapist who specializes in CBT.

PORTION DISTORTION

As you may have noticed in the EI questionnaires, people who focus a lot on calories tend to be more rigid in their dieting approaches. That's another reason I don't encourage calorie counting but rather a general awareness of high- and low-calorie foods. It's much simpler and more effective to simply eat less food.

Understanding portion distortion is far and away the single most important tool for learning how to eat less. A portion is how much food you choose to eat at one time, whether in a restaurant from a package, or in your own kitchen. If you teach yourself to identify a regular healthy-sized portion and routinely eat regular (instead of distorted) portions of food throughout the day, you could score an R every single day.

But for many people, determining a healthy portion size is downright confusing, for several reasons. The oversized portions now so common in prepared and restaurant foods (see the "Portion Distortion" table) lead people to believe that these jumbo portions are normal and therefore appropriate. Packaged foods list serving sizes, which may or may not be the same as what most people consider a portion. For example, a serving of Coke is 8 ounces (1 cup), but a can of Coke is 12 ounces, or 1½ servings. Likewise, a serving of pasta is a half cup, but most adults eat at least 1 cup of pasta at a meal, if not more. The same goes for breakfast cereal. As you'll notice in the sample breakfast menus in the Appendix, I recommend eating a full cup of dry cereal, which is technically 2 servings, if you go by the Nutrition Facts panel on the side of the box. Adding to the perplexity is the fact that some serving sizes are listed by weight rather than volume (that is, in ounces and grams, instead of tablespoons or cups), and sometimes they're listed as "dry weight," or "raw," or "uncooked." It's almost as bad as trying to count calories—who can keep track of all these different things?

Healthy Helpings: It's in Your Hands

Some nutritionists like to use objects like baseballs and ping-pong balls to help people visualize serving sizes. But that's not very helpful if you haven't seen a baseball up close since ninth grade. An even better tool for estimating a proper portion (or what I'll refer to as a helping) is with your hand. You can use your fist, palm, thumb, and thumb tip to estimate helpings for different types of foods (see "Hand-y Portion Sizes"). Chapter 6 includes more details about planning balanced meals with healthy helpings.

HAND-Y PORTION SIZES

Your Handy Guide for Portion Size!

1 thumb tip = 1 teaspoon of peanut butter, butter, or sugar

1 fist = 1 cup cereal, pasta, vegetables

1 handful = 1 oz. of nuts

1 finger = 1 oz. of cheese

1 palm = 3 oz. of meat, fish, or poultry

2 handfuls = 2 oz. of chips or pretzels

Source: A. Garner and J. Stuht. CORE tools and patient information: easy portion-control tips for reducing calories. *Obesity Management* 1(3): 113–115 (2005).

Smaller Snacks

Fortunately, some food manufacturers have bucked the supersizing trend and started offering smaller portion-controlled snacks, such as cookies and chips that contain just 100 calories. If you don't like buying snack packs, try making your own. When you buy a box of crackers, immediately portion them in plastic bags or containers. That way, they're ready to go when you need a snack. Although single-serving 8-ounce cups of yogurt used to be the norm, now you can buy 6- or even 4-ounce cups (the latter of which is the standard size in France). You can also buy 8-ounce mini-cans of cola.

PORTION DISTORTION

Food	Portion 20 years ago	Calories	Portion Today	Calories
Blueberry muffin	1.5 oz.	201	5 oz.	500
Bagel	3-inch-diameter	140	6-inch-diameter	350
Coffee drinks	8 oz. coffee (with whole milk and sugar)	45	12 oz. latte (with steamed whole milk and mocha syrup)	350
French fries	2.4 oz.	210	6.9 oz.	610
Fettuccine Alfredo	11 oz.	825	20 oz.	1,500
Pepperoni pizza	2 slices	500	2 large slices	850

Oversized portions are one of the prime reasons it's so easy to gain weight in America, as I explained in Chapter 2. As data from the National Heart, Lung, and Blood Institute shows, many everyday foods—from bagels to pasta dishes—have swelled in size, escalating their calorie counts.

NINE TIPS FOR EATING LESS

In addition to helping you avoid portion distortion, a number of other techniques can help you eat less throughout the day. Just as a leaky faucet will slowly but surely fill up a clogged sink, a constant trickle of a few extra calories every day piles on the pounds over time. Likewise, eliminating just a small amount of food from your daily fare will have the opposite effect. Below are some low-effort techniques to make that happen. Practice a new one every day for a week, then start adding them together. Eventually, they'll become part of your normal pattern.

1. Downsize your dishes

Serve your meals on smaller plates (on a salad plate, about 6 inches in diameter, instead of the usual 8- or 10-inch dinner plate) and you'll find it easier to eat smaller portions. See how the sphere on the left looks larger than the one on the right?

DOWNSIZE YOUR DISHES

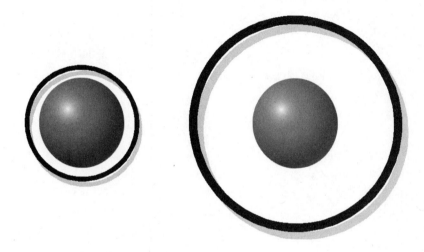

Likewise, a portion of food looks larger when served on a smaller plate than when on a larger plate. One study that involved eighty-five nutrition experts illustrates this point nicely. Each person got a small or large empty bowl and a small or large serving spoon. Everyone served their own ice cream and then filled out a brief survey while researchers weighed their ice cream. People given the larger bowls served and ate 31% more ice cream than those who got a smaller bowl. And larger scoops prompted people to serve themselves about 14% more ice cream. But everyone thought they had served themselves the same amount (about a cup) and were equally satisfied with their treat. Try the same technique at home and you'll never miss that extra amount. More details on plate management are in Chapter 6.

2. Leave one-eighth of your meals behind throughout the day

Remember how you divided your plate in quarters for the slow eating section? Just divide one of those quarters in half again to estimate one-eighth of your meal. Don't worry about precision—removing a few large bites is a close-enough approximation. This technique works with all types of meals and snacks. If you want to enjoy pizza or a hamburger with your family, just cut a small portion out and don't eat it. Likewise, carve a wedge out of your muffin or bagel. Place the extra food on a side salad plate before you start eating. It may seem like a strange habit at first, but it's very effective. Once you become skilled with this technique, you can adapt to serve yourself less in the first place.

3. Out of sight, out of mind

This is a subtle way to cut calories by making it easier to resist temptation. Make efforts not to stock your pantry with delectable high-calorie treats that beckon to you late at night. The success of this strategy depends on the family food shopper to make smart decisions at the grocery store. Leave that box of cookies or pint of ice cream on the store shelf. If it's not in front of you at home, you won't miss it. Follow this line of thinking in other aspects of your life by purposefully omitting food you don't need. For instance:

- Serve each plate in the kitchen instead of family style to lessen the temptation for taking second helpings.

- Stand away from the hors d'oeuvres or buffet table at a party.

- Take a detour on your way home from work to bypass the lure of fast-food restaurants.

In short, shield yourself from unnecessary cues and opportunities to eat.

4. Distract your appetite

Try eating a small snack, like a banana or a small handful of nuts, about a half-hour before your main meal of the day. Before going to a dinner party, social event, or holiday gathering, follow the same principle and "pre-eat" a sensible snack or mini-meal. That way, you won't be too hungry by the time you arrive at the event and will be less tempted by high-calorie party foods. The same goes for a trip to the grocery store: Shop after a meal or snack to avoid buying too much food.

5. Fill up with soup, salad, or fruit

Starting your meal with a broth-based soup, a green salad, or a piece of fruit can help you eat less. This strategy is based on the concept of energy density, which refers to the relative number of calories in a given amount of food. Low-energy-density foods contain lots of air, water, or fiber and tend to be low in calories. High-energy-density foods, such as meat, cheese, and fat, tend to be calorie-rich. Fatty foods tend to be very energy-dense, which is why a low-fat diet can help you lose weight; it's not because you're eating less fat but because you're likely eating fewer calories. By eating more low-energy-density foods like fruits and vegetables, you can eat a bigger volume of food, which helps you feel more full and satisfied than if you were to eat the same amount of calories from a high-energy-density food.

6. Share your restaurant fare

Most restaurant entrees contain far more food than a normal serving. For example, many dish up 4 to 6 cups of pasta or 16-ounce steaks. Share an entree, or ask the waitstaff to put half of your entree in a doggie bag at the very beginning of your meal so that you won't be tempted to pick at it. When dining at restaurants that pride themselves on large portions, try ordering just a side salad with an appetizer as your entree.

Before dinner, discuss your eating plan with your dining companions. Perhaps you'll encourage others to follow your lead.

7. Curb your choices at each meal

The wider the variety of foods available to you during a meal, the more food you'll eat. No doubt you've experienced this at buffets and potlucks. Numerous studies uphold this observation, like the one that found people ate more from a variety pack of jellybeans than from a single-flavor pack of the sweets. If you have just a few foods available at a meal, you'll eat those foods until you're full. You're less likely to overeat because eating more of the same thing isn't as pleasurable as eating something new—a phenomenon researchers have dubbed sensory-specific satiety. It's one of the reasons why single-food diets work well (but only for a short time, because that sort of rigid control will eventually lead to disinhibition). Sensory-specific satiety also explains why people often seem to have room for dessert, even if they're full. A second baked potato holds little appeal, but chocolate mousse is an entirely different story. Mind you, I'm definitely not saying you shouldn't eat a varied diet—quite the opposite. I encourage people to try new fruits, vegetables, whole grains, and seasonings to keep their diet tasty, fun, and interesting. Just curb the number of choices you have within a single meal so that you won't overeat.

8. Use a meal replacement

This tip is closely related to tip 7. Meal replacements such as Slim Fast, Boost, and Glucerna, which come as shakes or bars, make it easy to limit your choices and therefore trim the amount of food you eat. They're also very convenient and reasonably priced. What's more, meal replacements have been proven effective in aiding weight loss in a number of studies. But check the Nutrition Facts panel and you'll notice that most meal replacements contain around 220 calories—far less than the recommended 450. To help keep your hunger at bay, make sure you eat a small snack with your shake or bar, such as a piece of fruit or a small salad, along with a handful of pretzels or crackers.

9. Have breakfast for dinner

Here's another suggestion along the lines of the previous two tips. Eating a bowl of cereal for dinner is one of my personal favorites because it's so easy and tasty. In fact, Kellogg's and Post both promote eating two cereal-based meals a day as a proven weight-loss strategy. It's a great option for certain situations. For example, you had a very busy day and didn't have time to go shopping, or you had an evening meeting and didn't have time to prepare a full meal. Careful planning (which I'll describe more completely in Chapter 8) can help you avoid these time crunches. But you might find that you enjoy the simplicity and taste of having breakfast for dinner several times a week.

How can I tell if I'm eating less?

In addition to my presentations to colleagues and other professionals at meetings and conferences both in the United States and abroad, I speak at local community functions. At one of these engagements, a woman in the audience stood up and said, "I hear what you're saying and I'm trying to eat less, but how can I tell if I really am eating less?" Clearly, portion distortion has contributed to this confusion. But I told her that the answer is simple: Just step on your scale every morning. If it goes down, you're eating less!

SIX

Eat Well and Be Healthy

*What's really alarming is the major contribution of "empty calories" in
the American diet. We know people are eating a lot of junk food, but
to have almost one-third of American's calories coming from those
categories is a shocker.*

—Gladys Block, Ph.D.,
professor of epidemiology and public health nutrition,
University of California, Berkeley

GLORIA'S STORY: THE JUNK-FOOD JUNKIE

Gloria was a self-proclaimed junk-food junkie with a particular fondness for what she called the three C's: chocolate, Cheetos, and Coke. As
her three children were growing up, she grew used to having these
foods around the house. A busy family life left her little time to make
healthy meals, and it was easy to snack on those quick, filling treats.
Gloria was 5'6" and weighed 155 pounds—25 pounds more than what
she weighed before her first pregnancy. She came to our nutrition
clinic not only because she was worried about her weight but because
of her father. At 62, he was diagnosed with heart disease, and Gloria
was concerned that she might also be at risk.

Gloria's one-week food diary revealed an eating pattern that included several common violations. That made it easy to find places to
tweak her daily diet routine. Like many parents, Gloria was a victim
of kid-food syndrome, or eating a lot of foods normally targeted to
children. While getting her kids ready for school, she ate what she
served her kids for breakfast: a toaster pastry or a waffle. While packing their lunches, she rarely had time to prepare her own salad or
sandwich, so she often brought peanut butter and jelly sandwiches

(and Cheetos) for her own lunch, too. She brought fruit to snack on during the day but never missed her afternoon sugar fix of chocolate or cola.

Gloria had a tough time trying to convince her children to eat vegetables or whole grains, so family dinners consisted mainly of kid-friendly foods such as chicken nuggets, spaghetti and meatballs, and tacos. These foods are not particularly unhealthy in their own right (although deep-fried foods such as chicken nuggets should be a "sometimes" food rather than a regular meal). But the problem wasn't just what Gloria was eating—it was also about she wasn't eating. Because so many of her calories came from nonnutritious junk food, Gloria's diet was very low in several important nutrients, mainly vitamin D, calcium, and fiber.

Our plan was not to have Gloria make a drastic change but to make a slow, gradual transition toward a more healthful diet. These changes included eating more whole grains, ramping up her vegetable intake, and cutting back on the three C's.

Gloria and her kids did not like the nutty taste of whole grains, so she first switched to half whole-wheat, half white products. (Many types of bread, pastas, cereals, and some cookies contain whole-wheat flour, which is different than 100% whole wheat; see "Go for Whole Grains" later in this chapter for an explanation.) Her kids eventually made the switch from mostly refined breads and cereals to their 100% whole-grain counterparts, although they refused to eat whole-wheat pasta.

To boost her vegetable intake, Gloria swapped half of her daily Cheetos for baby carrots. She also treated herself to a prepared salad from the grocery salad bar once or twice a week. To sneak vegetables into her children's diets, she used tricks to make them more kid-friendly. For example, she gave them broccoli nachos made with low-fat cheddar cheese sauce, spinach dip on whole-grain crackers, and veggie-loaded baked potatoes.

Finally, Gloria bought portion-controlled servings of her other favorite treats—8-ounce cans of cola and "fun-size" chocolate candy bars—which helped her cut down on them. I suggested that she buy low-fat chocolate milk, which is a better choice than soda, for both herself and her kids. Over time, she incorporated even more changes and realized some key health benefits, as you'll see in the follow-up at the end of the chapter.

EAT MORE HEALTHFUL FOODS

Now that you've learned how to eat less, you're ready to move on to the next phase: eating well. Swapping some of the high-calorie processed foods you eat with fresh fruits, vegetables, and whole grains as Gloria did will reap both short- and long-term benefits. First, eating healthful foods allows you to eat bigger, more satisfying amounts, as you learned in the last chapter. It also makes it easier to spend twenty minutes

HEALTHY SUBSTITUTIONS: EAT MORE FOOD FOR THE SAME AMOUNT OF CALORIES

Instead of . . .	Try . . .
1 small bag of corn chips	1 small apple and 1 cup whole strawberries and 1 cup baby carrots with ¼ cup low-calorie dip
1 glazed doughnut	1 cup grapes and 2 apple cinnamon rice cakes topped with 1 tablespoon peanut butter
1 medium serving of french fries	1 small side salad with 2 tablespoons Italian dressing and ½ cup wild rice and 1 cup sugar snap peas and ½ cup raspberries with dollop of Cool Whip
1 chocolate croissant	1 cup Kashi cereal with 4 oz. skim milk ½ cup blueberries 1 hard-boiled egg

eating your meals, as I recommended in Chapter 5. Second, expanding your food repertoire can help keep your diet varied and interesting, so you'll be less likely to become bored or burned out. By creating a list of healthy foods that you like, you can easily prepare five basic meals that you can use every week.

You probably already know the long-term advantages of a healthful diet: lower rates of most health woes, from major killers such as heart disease, stroke, and cancer to less deadly but still debilitating conditions like cataracts, gallstones, and arthritis. Sometimes, it takes a health crisis—your own or that of a loved one, as was the case with Gloria—to be the tipping point that encourages you to change your eating habits. But whether you're worried about a current or future medical problem or simply want to make eating better more fun and tasty to help you lose weight and look better, this chapter will show you how.

COMPOSE YOUR PLATE

In the last chapter, you downsized your plate and portion sizes. Now, I'll show you how to upgrade the contents of your plate, based on the excellent New American Plate from the American Institute for Cancer Research (http://www.aicr.org). My variation on this theme sticks with the plate divided in quarters from Chapter 5, for simplicity's sake. Plus, you can use a plastic picnic plate with built-in separate sections (one large section and two smaller ones). Fill the large section with two or more vegetables. Make it a colorful mix, such as steamed broccoli and carrots flavored with a little olive oil, salt, and pepper, or a mixed green salad made with spinach or romaine lettuce. Then fill one small section with a whole-grain starch, such as brown rice or whole-wheat pasta, or a starchy vegetable, such as a baked white potato, sweet potato, or corn. Fill the last section with protein, such as grilled fish, chicken, or tofu. To create different versions, mix and match your own vegetable, starch, and protein from the table.

THE PRUDENT PLATE

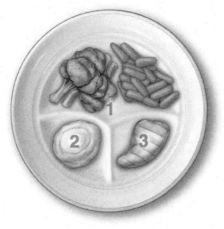

PLATE MANAGEMENT

Section 1 Vegetable (2 cups)	Section 2 Whole grain (2 oz. portion) or starchy vegetable	Section 3 Protein (3–4 oz. portion)
Asparagus Bell peppers Broccoli Brussels sprouts Carrots Cauliflower Cucumber Eggplant Green beans Kale Mixed green salad Spinach (2 cups cooked or 　4 cups raw) Squash Swiss chard Tomatoes	Brown rice (1 cup cooked 　or 2 oz. dry) Whole-wheat couscous 　(⅔ cup) Whole-wheat pasta 　(1 cup cooked or 2 oz. 　dry) Whole-wheat bread 　(2 slices) Corn (1 cup) Green peas (1 cup) Potato (1 medium or 1 cup 　mashed) Sweet potato (1 large or 　1 cup mashed)	Beans (1 cup) Beef, lean (1 small 　hamburger patty) Chicken (1 small breast) Eggs (2 eggs or 4 egg 　whites) Fish (1 salmon steak) Nuts (1 oz. = 24 almonds, 　14 walnut halves, 2 　tablespoon peanut 　butter) Pork (1 pork chop) Tofu (½ cup) Tuna (½ can [3 oz.] packed 　in water)

How does your plate stack up?

Think about what you had for dinner last night (or choose another of your typical dinners), and fill the blank plate on the left with the approximate amounts of each type of food you ate. How does your plate compare with the one I have suggested? Will your plate earn you an R, a K, or an O for the day?

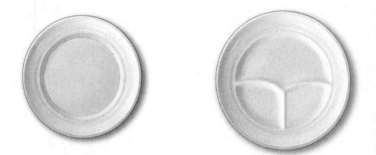

Now, consider how you might have tweaked your meal so that it reflects the eating well guidelines. Fill in the new amounts in the plate on the right. Try making that meal later this week.

BUILD YOUR PYRAMID

Let's step back and broaden the focus past the plate to your overall diet. To keep your diet interesting and healthy (two key factors to losing weight), heed the advice of the late David Kritchevsky, an internationally acclaimed expert on the role of diet in chronic disease. His counsel was simple: moderation, balance, and variety. You need a general sense of how much of each type of food you should eat, which will give you a better idea of how to stock your shopping cart and kitchen.

The U.S. Department of Agriculture (USDA) has been doling out nutrition advice for Americans for more than a century. The now-familiar

Food Pyramid, unveiled in 1992, organized healthy foods at the bottom, indicating they should form the base of your diet. Less healthy foods appear at the narrow top, to suggest you should eat only small amounts of them.

But nutrition science has evolved quite a bit since then. Not only has the USDA revised its pyramid but other experts have developed their own pyramids. My colleague, Walter Willett, M.D., a professor of epidemiology and nutrition at the Harvard School of Public Health, created the Healthy Eating Pyramid, which reflects the best of current nutritional science and resonates with my eating well principles.

THE HEALTHY EATING PYRAMID

What sets the Healthy Eating Pyramid apart from the USDA pyramid is how it distinguishes between different types of fats and proteins (plant-based versus animal-based) and different types of carbohydrates (whole-grain versus refined). Oils and fats found in seeds, nuts, and olives are more healthful than the type of fat found in meats and dairy. That's why plant-based fats appear in the second largest part of the pyramid, while red meat and butter are at the smaller top section. Similarly, whole-grain foods should be more common in your diet than white rice, white bread, and white pasta.

Note that daily exercise and weight control are at the base of the pyramid, which appropriately emphasizes their importance in resetting your set point. Next come fruits and vegetables, followed by nuts and legumes. Legumes—which include beans, peas, and peanuts—are all good sources of plant-based protein, as are nuts. Legumes are rich in fiber and other nutrients, which is why they're a good alternative to animal-based protein like fish, poultry, and eggs, which are located in the next level of the pyramid. Although nuts are high in fat, it is the healthy, unsaturated kind.

Dairy-based foods (milk, cheese, and yogurt) or a calcium supplement make up the next step. Because they are animal-based proteins, they contain more of the less-desirable types of fat, so choose low or nonfat versions of these foods. If you can't tolerate lactose, calcium supplements are a better option for you. The very top of the pyramid lists foods you should eat least frequently: refined starches, sweets, red meat, and butter.

Dr. Willett and his colleagues examined the diets of more than one hundred thousand adults while researching the Healthy Eating Pyramid. Men who followed the Healthy Eating Pyramid lowered their overall risk of certain diseases by 20%, compared with 11% for men who followed the original USDA Food Pyramid. For women, the comparable numbers were 11% and 3%, respectively.

One notable benefit to this eating style is that it's naturally low in salt, or sodium, which raises blood pressure in some people. The diet

THE HEALTHY EATING PYRAMID

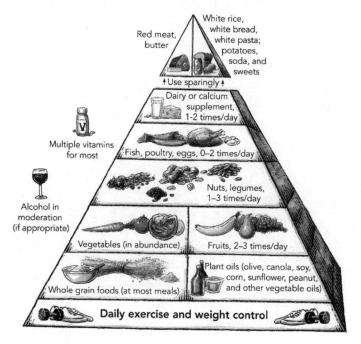

Walter Willett's Healthy Eating Pyramid advocates an eating style that reflects the best of current nutritional science.

GOOD SOURCES OF POTASSIUM

Food	Potassium (mg) in 1-cup serving
Bananas, raw	594
Cantaloupe	494
Potatoes, baked, flesh and skin	707
Prune juice	828
Spinach, cooked	839
Tomato products, canned, sauce	909
Winter squash	896

Source: National Heart, Lung, and Blood Institute.

is rich in key nutrients, namely potassium, but also calcium and magnesium—a mix of minerals that helps the body get rid of excess salt. If you have high blood pressure, this eating style can help lower your blood pressure—perhaps even as much as if you were taking medication, as one study has shown.

The Appendix includes four additional healthy eating pyramids that you may find more appealing or appropriate based on your food preferences (or age): the Vegetarian Pyramid, the Asian Pyramid, the Latin American Pyramid, and the Tufts Pyramid for Older Adults.

FOCUS ON FRUIT

Only about 25% of Americans eat the recommended amounts of fruits and vegetables, so it's clear that many people need some help adding these foods to their diet. Try these suggestions:

- Keep a bowl of fresh fruit wherever you spend the most time at home (in your kitchen or near your home computer, perhaps) to make it easy to grab a piece for a snack.

- Add fruit to your morning bowl of cereal (bananas, raisins, fresh or frozen berries) or to your lunch or dinner salads (chopped apples or pears, for instance).

- Keep a stash of small packages of dried fruit, like tiny boxes of raisins, at your workplace.

- Have a fruit smoothie for breakfast or a snack. Blend frozen strawberries, raspberries, or blackberries with low-fat milk or yogurt.

- Enjoy fruit for dessert, such as poached pears, baked apples, fruit sorbet, frozen fruit bars, or even chocolate-covered strawberries, in moderation.

- If you like canned fruits, look for brands with no added sugar or prepared in light or sugar-free syrup.

- Whole fruit is a better choice than fruit juice, but if you like a small glass in the morning, look for brands that contain 100% juice and no added sugar.

VARY YOUR VEGGIES

- A colorful salad for lunch or dinner is an easy way to boost your veggie intake (see the "Salad Suggestions" box).

- Keep plastic bags filled with carrot sticks, celery sticks, or other veggies in the fridge so that you can grab them for snacks and lunches.

- Frozen vegetables, such as broccoli, spinach, and corn, offer quick and convenient options for a dinner side dish. They're already washed and cut, and they won't turn limp or slimy before you can use them. Zap them in the microwave or thaw and sauté in a pan for a few minutes.

- Add vegetables to favorite recipes like spaghetti sauce, pizza, meatloaf, and stews.

- Pile tomatoes, lettuce, cucumbers, avocado, or other veggies on your sandwiches.

- Enhance the taste of vegetables with a pinch of salt or even sugar. Salad dressings, dips, or a little drizzle of olive oil can also boost flavor.

- If you like canned vegetables, look for low-salt or low-sodium brands, and rinse them before eating.

Do you have bad childhood memories of mushy canned spinach, bitter brussels sprouts, and bland iceberg lettuce salads? If that's your concept of vegetables, no wonder you don't eat them often. Simple recipes for tasty vegetable dishes, starches, and proteins, which you can use to mix and match to create your own healthy plates, appear in the Appendix.

GO FOR WHOLE GRAINS

Most people eat plenty of grain-based foods every day. But many of them are made with refined white flour, which is not as nutritious as whole-grain foods. Note that even if whole wheat appears on the label or the ingredient list, that doesn't mean the product is whole grain, because it may also contain white flour. Here are ways to take your whole-grain intake up another notch:

- When choosing bread, bagels, English muffins, and related foods, look for those made with 100% whole wheat in the ingredient list and make sure they contain at least 3 grams of fiber per serving (see "Nutrition Label Know-how" later in this chapter).

- For kids and others who balk at whole-wheat products, look for breads and other products made with white wheat, a different

Salad Suggestions

For a challenge, play the rainbow game. Make a salad with as many colors as you can: red tomatoes, orange carrots, yellow bell peppers, green lettuce and avocados, purple cabbage slices, white feta cheese, and black olives. You can even base your entire meal around a salad. Add leftover cooked veggies and grilled meat, fish, beans, hard-boiled eggs, nuts, or cheese for extra flavor and to make it more filling and satisfying. It's easy to do this by using the salad bar at your supermarket as Gloria did, but this can be expensive. As an alternative, provide your own salad basics from home (lettuce, peppers, cucumbers, tomatoes, carrots, onions, and dressing), and supplement with special items from the salad bar such as marinated veggies or olives. As you're building your salad, remember the plate management rule. A side salad should be all veggies, while a meal salad can have up to one-quarter protein (such as a grilled chicken breast, cooked garbanzo or kidney beans, or cubed tofu). And stick to a 1 tablespoon limit (about the size of half thumb) on the salad dressing to avoid going overboard on calories. (If you use low-calorie dressing, you can have 2 tablespoons.) Dried fruit and nuts can also add taste, texture, and variety.

variety of wheat that when milled closely resembles white flour, even though it's a whole grain.

- For cold breakfast cereals, good choices include Total, Cheerios, Grape-Nuts, Wheaties, Raisin Bran, wheat germ, granola, and Kashi 7-Grain Cereal. For hot cereals, try steel-cut oats, oatmeal, or oat bran (not Cream of Wheat or Cream of Rice). Like all your grains, cereal should have a minimum of 3 grams of fiber per serving.

- Use whole cornmeal for corn cakes, corn breads, and corn muffins.

- Snack on plain, lightly salted popcorn.

- Buy whole-grain pasta, or a whole-grain, part-white blend.

- Instead of white rice, try brown rice or other grains: kasha, quinoa, bulgur, wheat berries, whole-wheat couscous, or barley. Brown rice is now available in a quick-cooking form.

PICK YOUR PROTEIN

Just as with grain-based foods, Americans usually eat plenty of protein. The trick is choosing the leaner, healthier types of protein. Try adding more plant-based protein and trimming back on the amount of animal-based protein you eat. For instance:

- For beef, look for the leaner cuts, such as flank steak, sirloin tip side steak, eye round roast, brisket, and the leanest ground beef possible.

- Choose lean cuts of pork such as chops and pork loin. Avoid bacon, sausage, and cutlets.

- Select skinless white meat chicken. Beware of breaded, fried, battered, and/or processed chicken, such as chicken nuggets and patties, fried chicken, and chicken Parmesan.

- Ground turkey is a close taste substitute for ground beef. Fresh roast turkey breast is a good choice, as is sliced turkey in the deli section. Look for nitrate-free, low-sodium varieties.

- Try different varieties of fish, a great source of lean protein: salmon, snapper, cod, haddock, tuna, swordfish, mackerel, tilapia, sole, trout, and perch. Don't forget canned fishes such as tuna, salmon, and sardines. (See the "Supplement Savvy" section later in this chapter for more information about the importance of fish oil in the diet.)

- Soy products include tofu, tempeh, soy milk, soy yogurt, and soy cheese, as well as cereals enriched with soy protein (Kashi Go Lean Crunch and Quaker Weight Control Oatmeal).

- Boiled soybeans, or edamame, which resemble lima beans but with a different nutty flavor, are served in Japanese restaurants and are also sold frozen in supermarkets. You can eat these plain or toss them into a salad. Roasted soybeans, or soy nuts, are another good choice. Look for unsalted varieties.

- Many other beans are also great sources of both protein and fiber. You can buy many types dried (in packages or in bulk), but canned beans are real time-savers. Popular varieties include black, white, navy, pinto, and garbanzo (chickpeas).

- Like beans, nuts are another filling, healthful source of protein. You can add all sorts of nuts (almonds, pistachios, walnuts, pecans) to cereals and salads to add crunch and flavor. Watch your portion size, however, as nuts are high in fat and therefore calories. Stick to a small handful per day.

- Low-fat milk, yogurt, and cheese provide protein as well as calcium. Look for reduced (1% or 1.5% milk fat) or nonfat (skim) products.

- Eggs are an inexpensive, easy-to-prepare source of protein. If you have high cholesterol, don't have more than three or four per week, or simply toss out the yolks, which contain the fat and cholesterol.

MAKE OVER YOUR KITCHEN

Like Gloria and her family, most Americans eat a lot of junk food—about 30% of their daily calories, according to one study. For children or family members who demand these treats at home, or for cravings of your own, try the following steps to reduce junk food in your diet. Studies have shown that your taste buds will eventually adapt to prefer healthier foods and beverages.

- Cut down on the amount of junk food you buy each week. Start by buying one less bag of chips or cookies per week at the grocery store. If you drink soda, buy mini-cans.

- Make slow and subtle substitutions to replace junk food with healthier, more nutritious alternatives. For example, the whole-grain Fig Newtons or Chips Ahoy cookies could replace your favorite cookies.

- Don't deprive yourself. If eating one cookie per day will keep you from eating a bag a day, go for it (remember the dangers of disinhibition!).

- Repackage large bags of treats into single-serving snack bags and eat only one per day.

- Keep track of the number of times per day or week that you indulge in junk food in your R-K-O journal. Starting slowly, try to reduce the frequency by just one time a week. Notice that it's easier to score an R on the days that you don't eat junk food.

As Gloria's story shows, a single food shopper usually sets the tone for how the entire family will eat. Mothers sometimes worry that their kids eat too much junk food. But the truth is, they're usually in control of how much junk their kids eat. If Gloria simply stops buying toaster pastries, she and her kids won't eat them. If possible, don't take kids along when shopping, to prevent conflicts about what to purchase. But do encourage kids and other family members to help make the list so that they can add their own favorite fruits and other items. You might also agree to take turns choosing one special family snack such as one bag of potato chips or cookies each week.

Another important note about families: Studies show that the more often kids eat dinner with their families, the more likely they are to eat fruits and vegetables and the less likely they are to drink soda. Other research has found that kids who eat dinner with their families most days or every day are less likely to be overweight than kids who eat with their families less frequently. Making time for family meals has become more challenging in recent years, with the increasing numbers of working parents and kids with schedules packed with sports and other activities. Keep reading for suggestions on how to make frequent family meals more feasible. And check out Chapter 8 for tips on time management.

MEAL PLANNING

Once you clear out most of the junk, you'll need to restock. The secret to smart shopping is to plan meals and make a list. The Appendix has a list of basic provisions you should have on hand so that you can prepare healthy snacks and quick, easy-to-cook meals.

Planning a week's worth of meals may seem like a chore, but it can save you time in the long run. You should have a repertoire of at least five simple, healthy dinners that you can put together with little effort. If you're not a cook, try putting together a simple dinner using suggestions from the recipes in the Appendix. For example, you might have store-bought roasted chicken with a sweet potato and steamed broccoli, or baked or grilled salmon, brown rice, and roasted asparagus. Neither of these menus requires elaborate cooking, and they take only about thirty minutes to put together. If you already have a collection of favorite recipes, see "Recipe Checkup" (page 116) for tips on rating (and improving) the health of your recipes.

Cookbooks are a good source for menu-planning ideas. The upswing in the popularity of TV cooking shows over the past few years suggests that Americans may be more interested in making home-cooked meals. Some of these programs, especially those that emphasize healthy, lighter meals and/or kitchen shortcuts that minimize

Recipe Checkup

Can you tell if your favorite recipes qualify as healthful? In general, recipes that feature lots of vegetables (especially deeply colored ones such as broccoli, sweet potatoes, and peppers) are good bets, as well as those built around whole grains or beans. Cooking methods make a difference, too. For recipes that include meat, poultry, or fish, look for baking, broiling, roasting, or grilling rather than frying or deep-frying. And seek out recipes that call for unsaturated oils, such as olive or canola, instead of butter, shortening, or margarine.

You can also modify your recipes to lower the fat and/or boost the fiber. For example:

- When sautéing onions, garlic, and vegetables, use half the recommended amount of oil in a nonstick skillet.
- Substitute unsweetened applesauce or prune puree for part or all of the oil in recipes for baked goods, like muffins or quick breads, cakes or cookies. Try swapping one-third of the oil for applesauce to start, and then try one-half the next time to see what works best.
- Substitute up to half of the white flour with whole-wheat flour in recipes for baked goods (note that this may change the texture a bit).
- Remove the skin from poultry. Drain excess fat in the pan after cooking ground meat or after sautéing chicken, beef, or pork.
- Substitute vegetables for part of the meat in recipes for stews, soups, and casseroles.
- Use low-fat dairy products in recipes, substituting small amounts of more strongly flavored, full-fat cheeses like Parmesan or Romano to boost flavor.

Snack Packs

When you get home from the grocery store, set aside some ready-to-eat snack packs in small plastic bags or containers so that you can stave off hunger and avoid impulsive food purchases. Strategically place these snack packs in lunch boxes, in your purse, in your gym bag, in your car . . . wherever and whenever you think you might need a quick bite.

- Whole fresh fruit (apples, pears, oranges, bananas) or small cups of grapes, berries, or cubed melon
- Bell pepper slices, carrot sticks, or other veggies with prepared hummus dip or low-fat ranch dressing
- Carrot sticks, celery sticks, or apple slices with peanut butter
- Low-fat yogurt or cottage cheese cups
- Low-fat string cheese
- Hard-boiled eggs
- Whole-wheat crackers with peanut butter or cheese
- 100-calorie mini-bags of crackers or cookies
- Unsweetened applesauce cups
- Half of a small sandwich
- Whole-grain cereal or granola bars
- Small handfuls of nuts, trail mix, or dried fruit

preparation and cooking times, are definitely worth checking out. Also potentially helpful is the meal preparation franchise, such as Dream Dinners and Let's Dish, which are now available in many cities across the United States. These companies provide all the food and equipment you need to assemble a set number of dinners, which you then store in your freezer and serve over the upcoming weeks. Some offer healthy, lower-calorie options, provide nutrition information, and can be a less-expensive alternative to take-out or restaurant meals. If you don't have such an establishment near you (or want to be even more cost-effective), consider teaming up with several friends to prepare large batches of healthy dinners, either together or on your own time, which you can then swap with one another.

Once you've planned a week's worth of meals, make your list. No doubt you've heard the cardinal rule of food shopping: go to the store when you're fed and rested so that you won't be tempted to buy high-fat snacks or other treats. Another popular tip is to shop the perimeter, which is where you'll find the freshest, healthiest foods: raw produce, low-fat dairy products, fresh lean meats and fish. Venture into the interior aisles only when you're after specific foods such as pasta and canned beans, to avoid the temptation of chips, soda, and sweets. And make sure you look high and low; the foods at eye level are often some of the less-healthful items.

NUTRITION LABEL KNOW-HOW

If your local store doesn't feature a food rating system, the next best thing is to read the Nutrition Facts panel found on all packaged foods. Here's what you should pay attention to on the panel:

1. Calories: First, check the serving size and servings per container. How many servings will you eat? If you will eat more than one, be sure to multiply that number by the calories to determine the actual number of calories you'll consume. Does the calorie count fit into your meal goal of 450 calories?

2. Fats: Look for foods low in saturated fats, trans fats, and cholesterol to lower your risk of heart disease. For fat and cholesterol, low-fat is defined as 5% of the daily value or lower.

3. Sodium: Eating less then 2,300 milligrams of sodium (about 1 teaspoon of salt) a day may lower the risk of high blood pressure. Most of the sodium people eat comes from processed foods, not the salt shaker.

MACARONI AND CHEESE

Nutrition Facts

Serving Size 1 cup (228g)
Servings Per Container 2

Amount Per Serving

Calories 250	Calories from Fat 110

	% Daily Value*
Total Fat 12g	18%
Saturated Fat 3g	15%
Trans Fat 1.5g	
Cholesterol 30mg	10%
Sodium 470mg	20%
Total Carbohydrate 31g	10%
Dietary Fiber 0g	0%
Sugars 5g	
Protein 5g	

Vitamin A	4%
Vitamin C	2%
Calcium	20%
Iron	4%

* Percent Daily Values are based on a 2,000 calorie diet. Your Daily Values may be higher or lower depending on your calorie needs:

	Calories:	2,000	2,500
Total Fat	Less than	65g	80g
Sat Fat	Less than	20g	25g
Cholesterol	Less than	300mg	300mg
Sodium	Less than	2,400mg	2,400mg
Total Carbohydrate		300g	375g
Dietary Fiber		25g	30g

4. Fiber: When choosing grain-based foods (breads, crackers, cereal), look for products that contain at least 3 grams of fiber per serving. You should eat at least 25 grams of fiber per day.

5. Sugars: Sugar provides calories but few nutrients, so look for foods and beverages low in added sugars. Check the ingredient list to make sure that added sugars are not one of the first few ingredients. Other names for added sugars include sucrose, glucose, corn syrup, fructose, and high-fructose corn syrup.

6. Protein: Most adults should eat 60 to 70 grams of protein a day. Eating higher amounts (up to 100 grams) may help you feel full longer. Try eating a little extra protein if you find you're often hungry (but don't forget the 450 calories/20 minutes rule from the previous chapter).

7. Vitamins and minerals: Many Americans don't get enough vitamin A, vitamin D, calcium, and iron in their diet, so check this chapter to get a better sense of how the foods you eat contribute to your daily intake of these important nutrients. See "Supplement Savvy" for more information.

CONSULT A DIETITIAN

If you feel you could use some extra advice and guidance in changing your diet, meeting with a dietitian is a great idea. Registered dietitians (RDs) practice medical nutrition therapy and can provide targeted dietary advice for people with specific health concerns, such as diabetes or heart disease (including those at risk for these conditions, such as people with elevated blood sugar levels, high cholesterol, or high blood pressure). An RD can also help you to follow the eating well guidelines outlined in this chapter.

REVIEW YOUR RESTAURANT ROUTINE

Try to eat at home as much as you can. Home-cooked meals make it easier to control what and how much you eat and will save you a lot of money. But I realize that busy schedules, business meetings, and other circumstances (including happy ones, like a special anniversary or birthday meal, for instance) mean that most people will eat out at least once a week. Note that contrary to popular belief, your local bistro or neighborhood cafe isn't necessarily more healthful than a fast-food restaurant. In fact, sit-down meals can contain more fat, cholesterol, and salt than fast-food meals. Most restaurant owners have no incentive to serve healthy

High-Fat	Low-Fat
Au gratin	Baked
Breaded	Broiled
Buttered or buttery	Boiled
Cheese sauce	Grilled
Creamed, creamy, in cream sauce	Poached
Fried (deep-fried, french-fried, batter-fried, pan-fried)	Roasted
Gravy	Steamed
Hollandaise	Stir-fried
Parmesan	
Pastry	
Rich	
Sautéed	
Escalloped	
Scalloped	
Southern style	

food. Rather, they want to make sure their food tastes good and therefore sells well. That often translates into more salt, butter, oil, cream, and/or sugar than people cook with at home. And you already know the biggest problem with restaurant meals: the bloated portion sizes. Here are some suggestions for eating wisely away from home:

1. Plan ahead. Pick a restaurant that offers healthy choices. If you're not sure, call ahead to inquire. I helped initiate a program called Boston BestBites, a campaign to encourage restaurants to add or highlight healthy, light menu options; other larger U.S. cities are following suit. Try to scale back on how much you eat during the rest of the day, but don't skip a meal, because that will leave you ravenous and more likely to overeat. Have a small snack before you go out, or drink a large low-calorie beverage. If you want an alcoholic beverage, sip it with your meal, not before. If you're invited to a party, bring something healthy from home to share with others.

2. Choose carefully. Watch out for high-fat words (left column, above) on menus and look for lower-fat words (right column, above) instead.

Lower-Fat Choices	High-Fat Choices
Pizza Plain cheese pizza (ask for half the cheese or low-fat cheese) Onions, green peppers, mushrooms	Meat toppings (sausage/pepperoni) Olives
Burger place (fast food) Grilled, broiled, or roasted chicken without sauce Broiled extra-lean burger	Regular hamburger, cheeseburger French fries Fried fish or chicken Mayonnaise-based sauces
Mexican Heated (not fried) tortillas Grilled chicken or beef fajitas Soft tacos (corn or flour tortillas) Salsa	Enchiladas Chili con queso Fried tortillas, tortilla chips Sour cream, guacamole Crisp tacos
Chinese and Japanese Stir-fried chicken Stir-fried vegetables Steamed rice (ask for brown) Soup Teriyaki	Egg foo yong Fried chicken, beef, or fish Fried rice or noodles Egg rolls Fried wonton Tempura

Italian
Spaghetti with meatless tomato sauce
Minestrone soup
	Sausage
	Lasagna, manicotti, other pasta dishes
	    with cheese or cream
	Fried or breaded dishes (like veal or
	    eggplant Parmesan)

Seafood Broiled, baked, or poached seafood with lemon Plain baked potato	Fried fish Fried vegetables French fries
Steakhouses Shrimp cocktail Broiled chicken or fish Plain baked potato	Steak (except trimmed lean cuts) Fried fish or chicken Onion rings, other fried vegetables French fries

3. Ask for what you want, prepared the way you want. Order salad dressing, gravy, sauces, or spreads on the side, and request less or no cheese, if appropriate. Ask if foods can be cooked in a different way, and feel free to ask for foods that aren't on the menu. See if you can tweak your order so that you can compose your plate correctly; for instance, order a side salad or an extra side of vegetables and share an entree (or even a protein-based appetizer) with a dining partner.

Our staff dietitians who coach the participants in our diet studies encourage people to do role-playing exercises to practice talking with waitstaff. If you can have it your way at Burger King, you can certainly have it your way at a higher-priced restaurant. They recommend using a firm, friendly voice and looking the person in the eye. For example, if the waitstaff brings deep-fried fish, say, "This looks good, but I asked for my fish to be broiled. Would you have some broiled for me, please?"

4. Take charge of what's around you. Be the first person to order, which sets a positive example for the entire table. Keep foods off the table that you don't want to eat; for example, request "no bread basket, please." Ask that your plate be removed as soon as you finish.

SUPPLEMENT SAVVY: MULTIVITAMINS AND FISH OIL

Multivitamins

As I already explained, I'm not a fan of most dietary supplements, particularly those that (falsely) claim to enhance weight loss. And in general, I don't advise taking specific single-vitamin or single-mineral supplements. But like most nutrition experts, I recommend a daily multivitamin supplement for everyone. If you follow the eating well guidelines in this chapter, you'll probably get most of the recommended amounts of nutrients from food alone. In fact, many breakfast cereals contain most of the recommended daily intake (RDI) of important nutrients, because they're fortified with vitamins and minerals. Still, a multivitamin provides extra insurance for several key nutrients; namely, vitamin B_{12}, folic acid, and vitamin D.

Strict vegetarians or vegans need to be sure they get enough vitamin B_{12}, which is found naturally in meat and eggs. Also, many older people don't absorb B_{12} very well from its natural sources, but they can absorb the B_{12} added to fortified grains such as cereals and from multivitamins. Low levels of B_{12} can lead to anemia and neurological problems.

All women of childbearing age should take folic acid, another B vitamin, because it lowers the risk of birth defects. A multivitamin is also suggested for the same reason.

Multivitamins offer an easy way to make sure you're getting adequate amounts of vitamin D. This vitamin is important for strong bones, and a growing body of research suggests it may help fight prostate and other forms of cancer. Our bodies make vitamin D after being exposed to sunshine, but now that many of us avoid sunlight to spare our skin (from both wrinkles and skin cancer), many Americans are deficient in the sunshine vitamin. Since fortified milk and oily fish are the only important dietary sources of vitamin D, a multivitamin supplement can fill in the gap.

When choosing a multivitamin, buy a major brand name or store-brand product. When Consumers Union tested cut-rate products, it found that almost half didn't contain the listed amount of at least one nutrient.

Fish Oil Supplements

If you eat at least two to three servings of fatty fish such as salmon, albacore tuna, herring, mackerel, and sardines every week, you're reeling in the benefits of omega-3 fatty acids, the special heart-healthy fats found in fish. The evidence favoring these fats has been mounting for decades. Omega-3 fatty acids decrease the risk of rapid, unstable heart rhythms, lower harmful blood fats (triglycerides) in the blood, slow the growth of artery-clogging plaque, and even lower blood pressure a bit. People who eat fatty fish two to four times a week cut their risk of heart

BEST CHOICES FOR OMEGA-3s FROM FISH
AND SHELLFISH

Best Choices	Good Choices
Pollock	Canned tuna (light)
Salmon (fresh, frozen)	Shrimp
Herring	Cod
Atlantic mackerel	Catfish
Lake trout	Clams
Sardines	Scallops
Halibut	Lobster
Flounder or sole	Crab
Oysters	Grouper
Shark*	Mahimahi
Swordfish*	
Tilefish (golden bass or golden snapper)*	
King mackerel*	

Source: Modified from AHA Scientific Statement: Fish Consumption, Fish Oil, Omega-3 Fatty Acids and Cardiovascular Disease, 71-0241. *Circulation* 106 (2002): 2747–57.
*Highest levels of mercury (about 1 part per million Hg). According to the Food and Drug Administration, women who are pregnant, planning to become pregnant, or nursing, and young children, should not eat these fish. Everyone else can eat up to 7 ounces of high-mercury fish per week.

disease by about 30%. Those who don't care for fish or who don't have easy access to good sources of fish should take a daily fish oil supplement. Look for one that contains 500 milligrams of omega-3 fatty acids (often called DHA and EPA) per capsule.

GLORIA REVISITED

Over the course of six months, Gloria was able to gradually incorporate even more healthful changes into her diet. Instead of thinking of her new diet as cutting out all her old favorites, Gloria realized that she was taking a new approach that didn't leave her feeling deprived. For instance, she added more healthy substitutions, like swapping french fries with roasted nuts. She also switched from regular Coke to diet Coke and eventually to sparkling water. Gloria gradually made over her kitchen, replacing processed foods with fresher homemade meals. Knowing how to shop and having five recipes under her belt that were healthful, family-friendly, and simple to prepare were vital for Gloria and her family to make positive changes.

Gloria realized that these choices were becoming natural simply because they made her feel better. She could sense the difference in her clothes—her pants were no longer tight around her waist. While shopping for clothes, she realized she had actually dropped a size. She had more energy. After losing just a little weight, she could sleep more deeply and fall asleep much faster, so in the morning she was well rested instead of fatigued.

During a doctor's visit, Gloria learned that her systolic blood pressure (the first number) had gone down 10 points. Her cholesterol level had also dropped. Although Gloria came to us because she was worried about heart disease in her family medical history, she was astonished that her new habits and modest weight loss had such broad benefits, both for her immediate well-being and her long-term health.

SEVEN

Move More and Feel Great

There is no such thing as a good excuse for not exercising! If you look at your daily schedule, you can find some time to include exercise in your day. And once you do, you'll be amazed to find how energetic you feel afterwards.

—C. Everett Koop, M.D., Sc.D.,
former U.S. Surgeon General

Most Americans don't meet the national recommendations for physical activity, which call for thirty minutes of moderate exercise a day at least five days a week. Some say the environment in which we live is largely to blame for our sedentary ways. Long driving commutes, increased use of technology, and desk jobs, for example, make it easy to move very little. Consider Ned, for instance, who's a perfect example of the roughly 16% of Americans who are sedentary or inactive (defined as not engaging in any regular pattern of physical activity beyond daily functioning).

A DAY IN THE LIFE OF NED

- Ned awakens, gets ready for work, and stops at a drive-through doughnut shop for breakfast on the way to the office.

- He drives thirty minutes to work, munching his breakfast along the way, then circles his office parking lot for an extra five minutes to find the closest parking spot.

- Ned takes the elevator to the fourth floor, plops down at his desk, and hardly moves at all for another two hours. Everything—his computer, phone, and printer—are within arm's reach of his swivel chair.

- At 10:00 A.M., he walks a few yards to the office kitchen, gets another cup of coffee, and proceeds down the hallway to the meeting room.

- Two hours later, Ned and his coworkers take the elevator down two floors to the cafeteria, eat, and return back to their desks for an afternoon of sedentary office work and snacking.

- At the end of the day, Ned takes the elevator back to the parking lot, slides back into his car, runs some errands on the way home, and parks in front of his house.

- He then cooks and eats dinner, places the dishes in the dishwasher, moves a few feet into the living room, and settles down on his couch for some evening TV before heading up one flight of stairs to his bedroom for the night.

- Throughout the entire day, Ned manages to move very little, logging less than a mile's worth of steps, which classifies him as sedentary.

But you don't have to be like Ned. Consider Nancy, who faces the similar challenges of a modern suburban life. But she resists the temptation to rely completely on conveniences to do all her work and creatively adds short bursts of activity to her schedule throughout the day.

A DAY IN THE LIFE OF NANCY

- Nancy wakes and immediately takes her dog for a ten- to fifteen-minute walk, regardless of the weather. Afterward, she does fifteen minutes of stretching and calisthenics in her den while watching the morning news.

- Nancy drives to work, parks in the lot adjacent to her own building, and briskly walks to her office, which includes climbing six flights of stairs.

- Nancy avoids using the phone or email for correspondence that can be accomplished by talking to coworkers on the same floor.

- She also volunteers to be the office gopher, taking short breaks to run envelopes down to the mailroom or interoffice mail to other buildings.

- Instead of smoking or snack breaks, Nancy takes walking breaks and uses these fifteen-minute periods to circle her floor and perk up for the rest of the day.

- For lunch, she brings her own food and uses the extra time to take a walk outside or visits a cafeteria in a nearby building.

- Nancy stands at her desk whenever possible and finds that she's more alert with this extra movement.

- Once home, Nancy often visits the local store on foot (with her dog) to buy ingredients for dinner.

- She enjoys evening TV but uses commercial breaks to do laundry, make lunch for the next day, play with her dog, and move around. In any given day, Nancy doesn't sit still for more than twenty to thirty minutes at a time.

Physical activity is the third of the three key factors for resetting your set point, along with eating less and eating well. Although you can lose weight without boosting your activity level, the biggest challenge isn't the initial weight loss. The real test is maintaining that loss. And that's where exercise shines. Sticking to a regular exercise routine is one of the best predictors of weight-loss maintenance. Studies suggest you need at least one hour of exercise a day to keep off lost weight.

Exercise alone can't help you lose weight nearly as much as eating less. But doing both together, along with eating well, creates a synergy that will enhance your success.

Exercise: A Natural Appetite Suppressant

Contrary to what you might think, exercise helps curb your appetite. Your body's internal organs, such as the heart, lungs, and intestines, are controlled by nerves that work automatically. Because the nervous system controls involuntary actions, such as breathing and digesting, you're usually unaware of its activity. The autonomic nervous system includes two main systems. One controls the "fight or flight" response, which kicks in when you are under stress. Your heart beats faster, your pupils dilate, and blood is shunted away from your internal organs to your limbs, which allows you to run away from threats. The other system controls "rest and digest" functions—essentially the opposite of the fight or flight response. Your heartbeat slows and blood moves to the internal organs to help you digest and absorb food.

Your body can't activate both systems at once. Exercise activates the first system, while inactivating the other one. With the rest and digest system on hold, you feel less hungry, which is why exercise can actually help people eat less, as research has shown. If you have a tendency to eat most of your calories in the evening, try exercising before dinner to decrease your appetite a bit, which may enable you to eat a smaller or more healthful meal. Alternatively, consider taking a walk after dinner to deter yourself from eating dessert or a late-night snack.

Like eating well, exercising lowers the risk of heart disease, stroke, high blood pressure, and cancer. Regular exercisers are less likely to experience bone fractures, gallstones, Parkinson's disease, and ulcers. Beyond disease prevention, physical activity helps relieve stress, wards off depression, and can boost your immune system, which may lessen your chances of getting colds, the flu, and other minor illnesses. Exercise can help you sleep better, improve your sex life, and may even bring you a natural high by boosting your endorphins. In fact, many regular exercisers find that once they get in the groove, they feel bad when they don't exercise.

Finally, physical activity strengthens muscles throughout the body, including the heart. Sedentary people who start exercising soon notice that everyday tasks, like toting grocery bags from the car to the kitchen, take a little less effort. You may also find that climbing stairs and doing house and yard work become less strenuous and more enjoyable.

PHYSICAL ACTIVITY VERSUS EXERCISE

Before I walk you through the logistics of how to boost your activity level, let's start with some basic definitions. People often use the terms *physical activity* and *exercise* interchangeably. But technically, exercise is actually a subcategory of physical activity. Physical activity encompasses any movement that involves muscle contractions and an increase in metabolism. Exercise is planned or structured physical activity done regularly for the purpose of improving one or more aspects of fitness—aerobics, muscle strength, muscle–joint flexibility, or balance.

Types of Physical Activity

Experts further classify physical activity into groups based on the reason a person does the activity. For example:

- *Household physical activity* includes activities such as sweeping floors, scrubbing, washing windows, and raking the lawn.

- *Occupational physical activity* includes activities done as part of a person's job, such as walking, hauling, lifting, carpentry, shoveling, and packing boxes.

- *Transportation physical activity* consists of walking, biking, or similar activities to and from places like work, school, and stores.

- *Leisure-time physical activity* involves any exercise, sports, recreation, or hobbies that are not associated with activities related to any of the above three types of activities.

Another type of activity, known as *nonexercise activity thermogenesis*, or NEAT, has some overlap with the previous categories but also includes even smaller increments of activity, such as fidgeting, toe-tapping, and gum chewing (see the "Are you a NEAT-o-Type?" box).

Are You a NEAT-o-Type?

Do you know people who are always fidgeting or tapping and can never sit still? Chances are they are lean or at least leaner than their nonfidgety counterparts. Researchers have found that NEAT may be what separates lean people from those who are overweight. Lean people spend two more hours per day on their feet in NEAT, which is equal to about 350 calories of energy burned per day. It's easy to see how such a calorie difference could accumulate over time. In just ten days, 350 calories per day becomes 3,500 calories, which translates to about 1 pound of body weight.

The message is simple: if you spend most of the day in an office chair and are prone to couch potato tendencies at night, you need to move more. Fortunately, adding this type of movement isn't all that difficult, as long as you make a conscious effort not to sit absolutely still. If you have a sedentary job, try to get up and move around at least every thirty minutes during the day. Once you start this habit, it may become second nature. Try starting with the following:

- While you watch TV, stand or get down on the floor to do a few stretches.
- Better yet, scrap part of the evening TV and go for a walk after dinner.

(continued)

- Mow the lawn yourself using a push mower.
- Conduct "walking" meetings. Stand up when you're on the phone.
- Swap your office chair for a stability ball
- Be less efficient while doing household chores: alternate tasks on different floors so that you run up and down the stairs more often.
- Make extra trips down the driveway to get the mail and newspaper.

In short, find creative ways to increase the number of minutes you spend per day in NEAT and try to decrease the amount of time you spend sitting absolutely still. If you can add an hour of NEAT to the half-hour of recommended regular exercise you should get every day, you'll be well on your way to losing weight or maintaining your weight loss. The researcher who first described and continues to study NEAT, Dr. James Levine at the Mayo Clinic in Rochester, Minnesota, has designed an "office of the future" to increase NEAT throughout the day. His computer sits atop a specially designed treadmill that he walks on at a slow 1 mph rate while he checks email and talks on the phone. He conducts business meetings with coworkers as they walk around a "track" that envelops their office.

Types of Exercise

Exercise is also categorized by how it benefits your body and includes these groups:

- *Cardiorespiratory exercise* strengthens the heart and lungs. Examples include brisk walking, biking, jogging, or other exercise that increases your breathing and heart rate.

- *Strength training* (also called *resistance training*) builds muscle mass and strength. Examples include exercises that use weights, resistance machines, rubber tubing or bands, and calisthenics.

- *Flexibility training* encompasses all manner of stretching exercises, including yoga.

- *Balance training* consists of balance exercises such as tai chi, an ancient mind–body exercise from China that uses slow, gentle movements while standing,

How long and how intensely should I exercise?

The answer depends on your current level of fitness. If you haven't exercised in years, you'll need to start slowly. For some basic tips on getting started, see the table. It may take you several weeks before you reach the goal of doing thirty minutes per day. Keep in mind that, like Nancy, you can break up your exercise into ten- to fifteen-minute sessions.

HOW TO SAFELY INCREASE YOUR PHYSICAL ACTIVITY LEVEL

If . . .	Then . . .
Level 1: You do not currently engage in regular physical activity,	you should begin by incorporating a few minutes of physical activity into each day, gradually building up to thirty minutes or more of moderate-intensity activities.
Level 2: You are active, but at less than the recommended levels,	you should strive to adopt more consistent activity: moderate-intensity physical activity for thirty minutes or more on five or more days of the week, or vigorous-intensity physical activity for twenty minutes or more on three or more days of the week.
Level 3: You engage in moderate-intensity activities for at least thirty minutes on five or more days of the week,	you may achieve even greater health benefits by increase the time spent on those activities or the intensity of those activities.
Level 4: You regularly engage in vigorous-intensity activities twenty minutes or more on three or more days of the week,	you should continue to do so. Keep up the great work!

Source: Centers for Disease Control and Prevention.

What does moderate intensity mean? You can measure your pulse and do a little math or use a heart rate monitor to keep track of your intensity, but there's really no need to do so. Instead, just listen to your body. One simple method is the talk test: If you can carry on a conversation while you're exercising (you may feel a bit warm and may break into a light sweat), that's considered moderate intensity. If your breathing becomes heavy and talking becomes difficult or you can't finish sentences, that's considered vigorous intensity (see the table for examples).

Examples of Exercise Intensity Levels

Moderate-Intensity Activities

- Walking briskly
- Golf, pulling or carrying clubs
- Swimming, recreational
- Mowing lawn, power motor
- Tennis, doubles
- Bicycling 5 to 9 mph, level terrain or with a few hills
- Scrubbing floors or washing windows
- Weight training using machines or hand weights so that you don't exhaust the muscles

Vigorous-Intensity Activities

- Race walking, jogging, or running
- Swimming laps
- Mowing lawn with a push mower
- Tennis, singles
- Bicycling more than 10 mph or on steep uphill terrain
- Moving or pushing furniture
- Circuit training or weight training so that you are exerting great effort to complete the final few repetitions

(For a more detailed list, see the Appendix.)

Get Ready, Get Set . . .

Before starting any physical fitness program, make an appointment for a physical exam to identify any medical, physical, or mental limitations to exercise. Certain health conditions or physical limitations may affect the type or intensity of exercise you're able to do.

As I already mentioned, a pedometer can be a good way to track your activity level. Most people only log about 4,000 to 5,000 steps per day. For men, 1 mile is about 2,000 steps; for women, it's about 2,500 steps. I strive for at least 10,000 steps a day, which is the amount that studies suggest will help maintain weight loss. See Phase 1, Step 3, for more on getting started with a walking program. For help planning a walking or running route, sites such as www.gmap-pedometer.com that enable you to calculate the distance of your route can be helpful.

CREATING AN ACTIVITY ROUTINE

Create a schedule that is sufficiently flexible to accommodate your exercise sessions but rigid enough that you feel compelled to stick to your routine. That way, it becomes almost second nature. Here are other things to consider when planning your exercise routine:

Motivation: To help raise your motivation and accountability, don't go it alone. Find a walking partner (a person or a dog—your own pet or even a neighbor's) or a gym buddy. Join a group exercise class or hire a personal trainer, if you have the resources. It's harder to skip an exercise session if someone else is counting on you. Plus, it's nice to work toward a mutual goal with someone you like.

Early bird versus night owl: Figure out what time of day you prefer to exercise. Some people find that early morning workouts energize them for the day. Others like to relieve stress that builds during the day by exercising in the evening. Still others find they like to use their lunch break for a quick workout. In establishing your schedule and exercise routine, experiment with different times of day. Don't give up on exercising if you find it to be inconvenient or tiring—just choose a different part of the day that works better for you.

Empty stomach versus fully nourished: In the same way, people have preferences about how they like to coordinate mealtimes with exercise sessions. A full stomach can either interfere with a vigorous exercise session or provide the energy needed to complete it. Yoga, for example, is supposed to be practiced on an empty stomach. But if you're too hungry, you might not feel as though you have enough energy for a brisk walk or run.

Other preferences: Other issues may also affect the specific activity you choose.

- Do you like to sweat or not?

- What are your time constraints?

- What are your budget considerations?

- What other likes and dislikes will make you start and continue exercising?

PHASE 1: NEAT, STRETCHING, WALKING, CALISTHENICS

If you are sedentary (you don't exercise at all) or have taken an extended break from exercise because of an injury, illness, pregnancy, or time constraints, it's best to start by making small changes.

1. Add NEAT
The first easy change is to add NEAT to your daily activities by being creative and following Nancy's lead, particularly if you are prone to Ned's habits.

2. Add stretching to your daily routine

Try stretching for just ten to fifteen minutes when you first wake up, after you get home from work, or just before you go to bed. You can count these minutes as part of your total activity for the day. You don't have to follow any particular stretches, and you don't have to be flexible to feel the benefits of stretching. Stretching is a great beginning exercise because it will make you more aware of your breathing and more mindful of tight or flexible muscles in your body. And because it feels good, stretching can motivate you to try new physical activities, like walking. Just make sure not to overstretch. For a helpful guide featuring illustrations of different stretches and other exercise tips, I recommend *Exercise: A Program You Can Live With*, a Special Health Report from Harvard Health Publications (see Appendix for ordering information).

3. Add a short, brisk walk to your daily routine

Brisk walking is a great activity to start an exercise program, because all you need is a comfortable pair of walking shoes and a safe route. Not only is walking convenient (you can do it almost anywhere), it's also peaceful and can help relieve stress. With the booming emergence of portable music players such as iPods, many people find that listening to music, audio books, or Podcasts makes walking even more enjoyable. In fact, once you get started, it can become addictive. My wife, for example, can't function without her evening walk. She expends leftover energy from the day while working up a healthy, mild fatigue that ensures a good night's rest. Walking offers one of the most inexpensive ways to lose and maintain weight.

Start with just a ten-minute walk in your neighborhood or in a park every other day for a week. Gradually increase the amount of time you spend on each walk by one to three minutes a week and the number of times you walk per week. Use a pedometer to count steps if you prefer to measure distance instead of time. Pedometers motivate you to increase your steps. See how many minutes it takes to cover 2,000 to 2,500 steps, which is about 1 mile. Then, you can try to cover more distance in the same amount of time, or simply log more steps.

4. Add calisthenics to your weekly routine

Calisthenics are simple exercises that increase strength and flexibility using the weight of your own body for resistance. Some good examples to start out include crunches (modified sit-ups done with bent knees and toes tucked under the couch lip), modified push-ups (with knees instead of toes on the floor), stair climbing, and jumping jacks.

5. Combine

You may find more benefit from your stretching and walking routines when combined. Start with a five-minute warm-up walk, stretch for five minutes, pick up the pace with a brisk walk for ten minutes, do five minutes of push-ups and sit-ups, and conclude with five to ten minutes of stretching. In about thirty minutes a day, you can boost your health and strength. Give it a try and see how you feel!

6. Hobby

Many people have a hobby, such as gardening, hiking, or bird-watching, but don't make time to enjoy it. Thinking about ways to include more physical activity in your week is a good time to revisit the idea of joining a club or group of interest that will promote more physical activity in an enjoyable social setting.

Warming Up and Cooling Down

If you choose to skip the stretching routine, your exercise time should still include a warm-up and a cool-down period with at least a little stretching, to help prevent sore muscles. If you are older, you should spend a minimum of ten to fifteen minutes or almost equal amounts of time stretching as you do on other forms of exercising. Stretching helps protect your joints by maintaining their range of motion, allowing you to move more easily, and it may make injuries less likely.

PHASE 2: INCREASING MINUTES AND ADDING VARIETY

Once you achieve Phase 1 activity, keep building your weekly minutes and move on to Phase 2. If you are already meeting Phase 1 goals and consider yourself an intermediate exerciser—perhaps someone who likes to exercise but has never gotten hooked on it—then try the following suggestions to boost your weekly physical activity levels.

1. Add more steps or minutes

From your current daily step count, add 500 steps per week until you reach a goal of 10,000 steps per day. For example, someone accomplishing 4,000 steps per day in Week 1 might increase to 4,500 steps per day in Week 2 and 5,000 steps per day in Week 3, and so on. If you prefer to count minutes rather than steps, increase your daily time by one to five minutes per week in the same fashion, working toward a goal of thirty to forty-five minutes of physical activity per day most days of the week. (If you're curious about converting common exercise activities into steps, see the chart in the Appendix.)

2. Add variety to your routine

If you find your walking routine to be a little too monotonous, explore other physical activity options. For instance, try out some local hikes on the weekends or take a bike ride around a new neighborhood. And if you don't have a workout partner, exercise classes such as dance, kickboxing, and indoor cycling, led by an instructor and held at a local gym or studio, are a great way to spice up a stale routine. While it's important to stick to a relatively consistent exercise schedule, it's even more important to keep your routine fresh and interesting. Don't walk or run the same route every day. Try different exercise machines (treadmills, stair climbers, or stationary bikes) at the gym. Keep it challenging and exciting!

PHASE 3: STRENGTH AND RESISTANCE TRAINING PLUS MORE CARDIOVASCULAR EXERCISE

1. Add intensity (speed and/or resistance)

If you start at Phase 1, it will probably take a few months before you reach a moderately active or active physical activity level. When you reach this activity level, you may not have time to add more minutes to your fitness schedule. Another effective way to get stronger and burn more calories is to increase your intensity, particularly during cardiovascular exercise. In general, think of increasing intensity by increasing speed, resistance, or both at once:

- If you have healthy knees and joints, you might want to try ramping up your brisk walk into a slow jog or run.

- Incorporate a few fifteen- to twenty-second high-energy efforts or sprints when walking, jogging, biking, rowing, swimming, or using cardio equipment at the gym.

- Incorporate stair climbing, small hills, and/or resistance into these activities. (With swimming, you can use hand paddles to increase drag.)

- Partner up with a friend and add some healthy competition to your routine. Race for short intervals; challenge each other to push harder.

2. Cross training

Cross training, which means performing a variety of different activities and/or sports, has both mental and physical benefits. For your brain, the variety and new challenges keep you engaged and interested. For your body, cross training helps correct the lopsided physical effects of doing only one type of exercise. For example, running is a great exercise for your heart, legs, and mind. But it doesn't do much for your upper body strength and tone. Runners are prone to have tight hamstrings (the muscles that run up the back of the legs) and lower back muscles but well-developed quadriceps (the muscles on the front of the legs). Therefore, a jogger could cross train by lifting weights and attending yoga or stretching classes a few times per week to even out the effects of running.

3. Strength training

Strength training, also known as resistance training or weight training, consists of weight-bearing exercises that make the muscles work harder than usual. This added effort causes the muscles to get stronger. Contrary to popular belief, you don't need fancy equipment to practice strength-

---

What and How Much to Drink When Exercising

Most people don't drink enough fluids during or after exercise. For any exercise that raises your heart rate, the rule of thumb is to drink 1 ounce of water for every minute you work out. So if you spent forty minutes on the treadmill, you would need two 20-ounce bottles of water. Most of the time, plain old water—maybe with a lemon or lime slice or splash of juice for added flavor—is a good choice for the average workout.

Sometimes, energy drinks like Gatorade or Powerade make sense. For example, during exercise that lasts more than an hour, such as a long bike ride or a hike, you may need energy drinks to avoid feeling weak or tired. These drinks contain water, carbohydrate (sugar), minerals, and electrolytes (salts). The sugar provides an energy boost to your muscles, while the salts replenishes substances you lose in your sweat. The salt also helps your body absorb and hold onto water, triggering your thirst mechanism and encouraging you to drink more. But beware of the calories: a 32-ounce bottle of Gatorade has 200 calories, which most people don't need unless they're really exercising intensely. You can also dilute the beverages (three parts water to one part energy drink), as many athletes do, or look for a low-calorie version or flavored water.

training exercises. Push-ups, pull-ups, and sit-ups are all weight-bearing. You need to do these exercises correctly to avoid hurting yourself, which will probably require some help from an instructor. This is especially true when you are ready to move up to free weights (small handheld dumb-bells or wrist or ankle weights) or to use resistance-training machines in a gym. In-person demonstrations from trainers/coaches/trained friends are the best. Exercise videos are also fine, provided you are careful and follow directions to perform the exercises correctly.

Strength training increases lean muscle mass, which can help you burn calories faster and can make bones denser, which protects against osteoporosis. It's also a great way to add variety to your exercise routine, and the results—all of the above, plus a more toned body—are very satisfying. Another report from Harvard Health Publications, *Strength and Power Training: A Guide for Adults of all Ages,* is a good source for il-lustrated instructions for strength training (see the Selected Resources).

WORKING OUT WITH OTHERS

While some people prefer to exercise alone, others find that group ex-ercise makes exercise more fun and boosts motivation. You don't have to join a health club; many communities offer a variety of different classes at different venues, including:

- YMCA, YWCA, JCC
- University or high school recreational centers that offer public membership
- Adult community centers and education classes
- Boys' and Girls' Clubs (some offer adult classes, too)
- Senior centers
- Independent yoga and fitness studios
- Classes at local dance studios

You can exercise at public pools, tennis courts, basketball courts, ice-skating rinks, and tracks. Also, some hotels allow nonguests to use their exercise facilities or swimming pools for a fee, which can be a good option if you work nearby and can go before or after work. Finally, inquire at your workplace about fitness-related benefits, which may extend to your entire family. You may be able to get a lower corporate rate at a local health club or gym, or use on-site athletic facilities if you work in an academic environment.

Other Group Exercise Ideas

- Join a neighborhood/community intramural team, like an office softball team.

- Create a neighborhood or office walking group.

- Try exercise videos at home with family or friends.

- Get a small group of friends together and inquire about group rates with a trainer to lower the expense.

- Join a local cycling club.

Recommended Classes
(especially for beginners and older people)

For people new to exercise or who want a gentler, less intense workout, the following types of classes are a good bet. Each type offers broader benefits and can help balance out any exercise routine, no matter what your fitness level. For any class you take, it's very important to find a qualified instructor. Ask if the instructor is certified to teach his or her particular specialty, and listen closely to what the instructor says during the first class. Good instructors will ask if you have any health issues that may affect your ability to do the specific exercise (not just a medical condition but a bum knee or bad back, for example), and they will also stress that you listen to your body and not push yourself too hard, despite what others in the class may be doing.

Yoga: To build flexibility, boost strength, promote relaxation, and possibly help you keep off weight, consider taking a yoga class. A two-year study of more than one thousand adults in their mid-50s who did yoga regularly found that the practice helped attenuate weight gain, especially among people who were overweight. As the study authors note, most forms of gentle Hatha-style yoga (as done in this study) don't provide enough moderate-intensity exercise to explain the weight-related effect. Rather, they believe the effect may be due to the fact that people who do yoga regularly feel more connected to their bodies and have a sense of well-being that helps them avoid junk food and overeating. There are many different forms of yoga, ranging from Hatha yoga to more vigorous, sweaty forms, such as Ashtanga or power yoga. Be sure to start with a class intended for beginners. If you choose, you can then move on to a more challenging class when you're ready.

Tai chi: This ancient Chinese form of exercise involves gentle, flowing movements linked together by breath. Many studies show that this type of exercise benefits older people in particular because it improves balance, which can lower the likelihood of falls. Tai chi also strengthens the legs; increases the range of motion of the shoulders, wrists, knees, and ankles; and improves posture. People say the exercises help them feel calmer and less stressed.

Water aerobics (Aquacize) and other exercises: Done in a swimming pool in waist-deep or chest-deep water, this form of exercise has the advantage of exercising all your muscles and joints without fighting gravity, thanks to the buoyant effects of water. Water aerobics can increase your heart and breathing rate but keep you cool so that you don't sweat. The buoyancy makes it a little easier to stretch and lengthen your muscles. The Arthritis Foundation has developed a water-based program for people with arthritis that is appropriate for anyone who would like to start an exercise program. The program provides supervision of safe exercises in a supportive social environment. Contact the local chapter of the Arthritis Foundation for more information (see the Selected Resources).

> ### American College of Sports Medicine
>
> Another excellent source of information on exercise, health, and fitness is the American College of Sports Medicine (full disclosure: I'm one of the founding members). The ACSM works to spread the benefits of physical activity. They provide free brochures to the general public, many of which can be downloaded from the Web, which describe how to choose and effectively use a wide range of different types of fitness equipment, from stability balls to free weights to exercise bicycles (see the Selected Resources).

TRACKING YOUR PROGRESS

It's a good idea to track your exercise progress with an activity log, or at the very least, take a few minutes once a month to consider how you're doing fitness-wise. Seeing your progress can be motivating. Take a reading before you start so that you have a basis for comparison. The following are standard physical activity tests to monitor your improvement and effort levels.

Track Test

For this test, you can either measure time over a certain distance or measure distance in a certain amount of time. Take advantage of a nearby track at a local high school or college. See how long it takes you to walk a quarter of a mile (one lap around a standard track) or run/walk 1 mile (four laps). Redo this test monthly as you build your endurance to see if you can beat your original time.

Alternatively, you can use a pedometer to measure distance in terms of steps. Give yourself a time parameter of fifteen minutes. See how much distance (number of steps or laps around the track) you can cover in fifteen minutes. Again, return to this test monthly and see if you can beat your original distance. If it usually takes you fifteen minutes to walk a brisk mile, then you can use your watch and pedometer as extra motivators on days that you feel like you are dragging somewhat. If you don't have access to a track or prefer to exercise indoors, both of these tests can be performed on either a treadmill or stationary bike. Ideally, the machines will have a measure of distance traveled so that you can record and compare your progress from time to time.

Six-Minute Walking Test

The six-minute walking test is an alternative measure that may be a better choice for people who are less active, older, who have a chronic disease, or who are less fit. Like the track test, the goal is to cover as much distance (on a track or hallway) as possible within six minutes, without running. Wear comfortable shoes and clothing and rest or stop when necessary.

Heart Rate Monitor

Once you get to an elite level, a heart monitor offers a great way to assess your overall effort. Most monitors have a chest strap with a wristwatch that shows your heart's beats per minute (bpm), or pulse. Everyone has a maximum heart rate, based mainly on age, gender, fitness level, and genetics. Heart rate monitors can also help gauge your effort. Say you're really tired one day and notice that you are only working at 50% of your heart rate. You can ramp up your effort to increase your heart rate, or you can try again on a day when you are better rested. Like pedometers and stopwatches, heart rate monitors are just tools that bring awareness to your physical activity level and progress.

PLAY IT SAFE: AVOID
EXERCISE-RELATED INJURIES

Some people assume that most exercise-related injuries occur in professional athletes or weekend warriors who don't work out regularly and then overextend or overstress themselves during a long, intense exercise session. But most injuries actually occur from cumulative microtrauma, or continued wear and tear on a particular tendon, joint, or muscle.

One of the most common exercise-related injuries is tendonitis, which is swelling and pain in a tendon, the tissue that connects muscle to bone. Some common sites include the shoulder (rotator cuff, from swimming), elbow (epicondylitis, from golf or tennis), and ankle (Achilles tendon, from jogging or running). Runners and even serious walkers may experience shin splits, caused by tiny tears in the muscles that attach to the shinbone. Warming up and stretching can help prevent these injuries, as can proper footwear, in the case of shin splints. Another great way to avoid injuries is to vary your exercise routine so that you don't put so much wear and tear on the same part of your body.

When starting a new exercise routine, you may feel stiff and sore for the first day or so. That's normal. But how can you tell if you've gone too far and hurt yourself? Diffuse muscle pain and soreness can last up to seventy-two hours after a strenuous workout. But if your discomfort persists longer than that, you may have injured a muscle or other structure and should see your doctor for advice. If you feel very sore or stiff a day or two after you exercise, you may be pushing too hard. Cut back on the time and intensity of your exercise and then gradually build up.

Depending on your injury, your doctor may refer you to a physical therapist (PT), who can help ease the swelling and pain with therapeutic exercises or hands-on therapy, and can also teach proper exercise technique and form. According to the American Association of Physical Therapists, many people unknowingly contribute to their own pain by exercising improperly or with poor posture. A physical therapist can identify and correct those problems. Note that in some (but not all) states, you need a referral from your physician to see a PT.

EIGHT

Synchronicity: Time, Sleep, and Weight Loss

Clearly, sleep is not only for the brain but also for the rest of the body. Recent evidence suggests that sleep loss, a highly prevalent—and often strongly encouraged—condition in modern society could be a risk factor for major chronic diseases, including obesity and diabetes.

—Eve Van Cauter, Ph.D.,
University of Chicago

BARBARA'S STORY: SMOOTHING OUT A TIME CRUNCH

A mother of two young teenagers, Barbara worked full-time, commuting more than an hour each way to her office. On a typical day, she would rise around 6:00 A.M., spend the next hour and a half getting ready for work, making coffee and a quick breakfast while coaxing her kids out of bed and making sure they had everything they needed for school and extracurricular activities. She left home around 7:30 A.M. and walked two blocks to the commuter train station, usually arriving to work around 8:45 A.M. Her husband drove the kids to school.

Barbara never found time to take a lunch break. Instead, she would snack at her desk throughout the day. She tried to leave by 5:00 P.M. to get home by 6:00 or 6:30 P.M., when she would pick up her kids from their after-school activities, sometimes chauffeuring them to another lesson or activity. Barbara's family valued their weeknight dinner ritual, but time constraints often led her to rely on quick and sometimes unhealthy shortcuts. Dinner and cleanup were usually done by 8:30 P.M., when her kids did homework and she and her husband spent time catching up. They usually stayed up until 11:30 P.M. to watch a 10:00 TV show and the 11:00 news together. Weekends were equally busy for Barbara, between caring for her elderly grandmother, shopping for groceries, doing laundry, running errands, and escorting the kids to their activities.

Like many middle-aged moms, Barbara spent so much time caring for everyone else that she rarely had time for herself. She was unhappy with her weight and her fitness level, but she truly didn't have the time to squeeze anything else into an already hectic week. Upon her 50th birthday, she decided it was time for a big change. But she needed support from her coworkers and family.

First, she looked into changing her work schedule. To minimize her weekly commuting time, she asked to work four 10-hour days, Monday through Thursday from 7:30 A.M. to 5:30 P.M. She gained time by cutting the Friday commute and avoiding the worst part of rush hour on the other days. As a veteran employee at her company, she was granted this schedule change without much hassle. Barbara also managed to carve out a fifteen to twenty-minute lunch break for a salad or leftovers. She and her husband gave up their 10:00 P.M. TV show. Because they were naturally early risers, the earlier bedtime and 5:00 A.M. wake-up suited them nicely. They slept seven hours per night during the week and eight to nine hours on the weekends. Her husband still drove the kids to school Monday through Thursday, and she picked up the slack on Friday.

Having Friday free was the payoff for a busy week. She did all of her grocery shopping on Friday morning when the stores were quiet. Barbara also used this day to visit and assist her elderly grandmother. On Friday afternoon, she dedicated two hours to her health. She set up their old treadmill in her basement and walked on it for an hour, often multitasking this with laundry and other housekeeping. Later, when this routine became mundane, she joined a local gym. She also started going to Weight Watchers with her two sisters.

Barbara did high-intensity or longer-duration exercise on the weekends when she had more time and was more rested. After-dinner walks sufficed during the week. She dedicated Saturday and Sunday to family activities, like football games and recitals. She and her husband taped weeknight TV shows and watched them on Friday and Saturday evenings when the kids were out with friends. Sunday afternoon, when the kids did homework, she planned and cooked many of the meals for the week. For example, Sunday dinner usually included grilled or roasted meat and vegetables, some of which could be saved for a pasta dish on Monday. She would assemble a healthful casserole to bake on Tuesday night, and leftovers could be eaten on Wednesday. Thursday night was reserved for carry-out and/or quick frozen dishes.

Barbara's strong organizational skills and her early-bird tendencies allowed her to continue her caretaking tasks while also caring more for herself. She gained quality time with her kids on the weekends and Friday afternoons. Figuring out a workable schedule took some time and experimenting, but her dedication to the program enabled her and her family to eat well, be physically active, and enjoy their time together. Though Barbara's schedule wouldn't work for everyone, it works for her. This chapter will help you find ways to create your own time-efficient schedule.

MAKING TIME TO CHANGE

One of the most important yet often overlooked aspects of losing weight and staying healthy is using your time efficiently. There's no getting around the fact that making the commitment to lose weight takes time. You need time to rest and to exercise, as well as time to shop for, prepare, and eat healthful food. But when people say they don't have enough time to do those things, that's not strictly true. They're simply choosing to spend their time doing different things. Setting priorities is a major part of changing your habits. The improved quality of life you can realize with effective time management is often the tipping point for a healthy living makeover.

An irregular, disorganized schedule interferes with good sleep hygiene. Getting enough sleep on a regular basis ranks at the top of my time priority list, as you'll see from the emphasis on sleep in this chapter. Your body and mind need plenty of rest to exercise and function well throughout the day. More importantly, insufficient sleep raises the risk of being overweight and developing related problems such as diabetes, heart disease, and certain cancers.

By taking a closer look at exactly how you spend your time every day, you'll gain a better appreciation for how much free or discretionary time you actually have. Then, you can experiment with simple time-saving tips that will help you develop a regular schedule and add healthy habits to your daily routine.

NEVER SACRIFICE SLEEP

When planning the best way to allocate your time, sufficient sleep should be your number one concern. One of the biggest mistakes busy people make is staying up too late or getting up extra early to get more things done. That strategy can backfire, especially if you're trying to lose weight.

On average, most adults need seven to nine hours of sleep per night. Some people need a little more, some a little less. And most of us don't get enough. A 2005 poll by the National Sleep Foundation (NSF) reported that 40% of those interviewed get less than seven hours of sleep a night. Think of your sleep time as a necessity rather than a luxury. Contrary to conventional wisdom, the need for sleep doesn't decline with age, although it may become more difficult to get all your sleep during a single uninterrupted time period. If you can't get at least seven hours of uninterrupted sleep a night, a brief (no longer than forty-five minutes) daytime nap can be a good way to get some extra shut-eye.

You'll know if you slept enough by how you feel when you wake up in the morning. Do you feel rested and energetic? If not, try going to bed a little earlier. In our time-pressed world, it's easy to sacrifice sleep to make more time for work or play. But if you're not well rested, you won't be as effective during the hours you're awake, which can waste time over the long run. In fact, the NSF poll revealed that 28% of the

Napping 101

If you're among the many people who get fewer than seven hours of sleep a night, short daytime naps can be a good way to catch up. While some people love naps, others find naps challenging—either they can't drop off easily, or they feel too groggy and disoriented upon waking. It turns out that there are good naps and not-so-good naps. If you're short on sleep (you stayed up too late worrying about work or had to soothe a wakeful child, for instance), a twenty- to thirty-minute snooze in the early or midafternoon can pep you up. (Of course, this may not be feasible on weekdays for those who work, but weekends can be a good bet.)

But if you nap too late in the day or stay asleep too long, you may have trouble falling asleep at night, which can perpetuate a bad cycle. Note that if you awaken from a nap feeling groggy instead of refreshed (usually because you slept too long), you may need to simulate your morning wake-up routine to get going again. For example, taking a shower or doing a quick burst of exercise (a brisk walk, stretching, or calisthenics) can help.

respondents said they missed work, events, and activities or made mistakes at work in the prior three months due to inadequate sleep or sleep problems. If you feel lethargic from lack of sleep, you'll be less likely to muster the energy to exercise. Fortunately, being physically active peps you up during the day but creates a healthy fatigue at night, which can help you sleep better. Again, the synergy of the set point solution works in your favor.

SLEEP SHORTAGE, WEIGHT SURPLUS

The main reason sleep is so vital to resetting your set point stems from a growing body of research showing a close link between duration of sleep and body weight. Research shows that middle-aged adults who sleep less than eight hours a night are more likely to be overweight. The less sleep you get, the more likely you are to be overweight. In fact, sleeping only four to five hours a night increases your likelihood of being obese by 50% to 73%. The Harvard Nurses' Health Study of more than sixty-eight thousand women found that women who slept seven to eight hours were the least likely to experience a major weight gain over the sixteen-year follow-up. Women who slept six or fewer hours per night had a 12% higher risk of gaining 33 pounds. But those who slept five hours or less had nearly a one in three chance of gaining 33 pounds. And more than a dozen studies of children, including those ranging from age 3 to 18 years, have documented a link between insufficient sleep and a higher body weight.

The Science Behind Sleep Loss and Weight Gain

Experts have many different theories about what drives this trend. For one, people who sleep less are awake longer and therefore have more opportunities to eat. Second, sleep affects the hormones that regulate feeding and appetite control. Researchers have found that sleep-deprived people secrete more ghrelin, a hunger-inducing hormone. Overtired people may also be in a state of high alert during the day, producing more stress hormones like adrenaline that can be harmful to a person's health over time. These hormones may boost appetite and a desire for high-calorie food, which may explain the pizza cravings of college students who pull all-nighters. Feeling tired makes you more prone to disinhibition: you're too exhausted to seek out a healthful choice, so you just eat whatever's available.

As mentioned in Chapter 1, the hypothalamus helps regulate not only hunger and eating behavior but also sleep–wake cycles. This is not a coincidence. After all, animals need to be able to adapt their sleep–wake cycles to their environment so that they'll be awake and active when food is available. Research suggests that disrupting the normal sleep–wake cycle—for example, not getting enough sleep—can have negative effects on eating and exercising habits.

For your health, body weight, and sanity, getting enough shut-eye may be your first line of defense against weight gain and chronic disease. Think of sleep as one relatively simple and pleasant lifestyle change you can make toward attaining a healthy weight. After all, who doesn't love sleeping well and feeling rested? For my patients who say they've failed in their earlier efforts to lose weight, my first question is: What time do you go to bed? And my first recommendation is: Early to bed, early to rise.

OVERSTIMULATION: A COMMON CAUSE FOR UNREST

Why are people often short on sleep? Time pressure, or feeling the need to get everything done, is perhaps the biggest culprit. Overstimulation— usually the result of too much screen time from both television and computers—is also a factor. Stimulants like caffeine and nicotine only make the problem worse. Certain people tend to be more vulnerable to sleep deprivation, such as students, shift workers, and travelers, as well as those suffering from acute stress, depression, or chronic pain. For these people, sleep schedule adjustments can be especially challenging. The same is true for people who work long hours or multiple jobs, as well as new parents dealing with an infant's erratic sleep schedule.

The NSF and other sleep experts recommend not eating, drinking, or exercising within a few hours of bedtime. But remember to stay flexible and find a balance that suits your lifestyle. It's true that for some people, eating a heavy meal in the evening may trigger sleep-disrupting heartburn or indigestion. And drinking any type of fluid too close to bedtime might cause you to awaken to use the bathroom. But when it comes to eating, timing matters far less than amount. If you find that a small snack or glass of low-fat milk close to bedtime helps you nod off, that's great—don't stop. Listen to your body and do what works for

Shut-Eye Solutions

To get into a good sleep schedule, follow this advice from the National Sleep Foundation:

1. **Make every effort to go to bed and wake up at the same time every day, including weekends.** This helps set your body clock, helping you fall asleep at night.
2. **Follow a regular, relaxing bedtime routine**. Taking a hot bath, then reading a book or listening to soothing music, can help ease you into a sounder sleep. Avoid stimulation from arousing activities (like working or paying bills) and bright lights, which can make falling and staying asleep more difficult.
3. **Create a soothing sleeping environment.** Sleep on a comfortable mattress and pillows in a pleasant, dark, and quiet room.
4. **Use your bedroom only for sleep and sex.** Keep work materials, computers, and televisions out of the sleeping environment to avoid possible distractions.
5. **Avoid caffeine (in coffee, tea, soft drinks, and chocolate) in the late afternoon and evening.** Caffeine's stimulating effects usually last three to five hours, but for some people, they may linger for twelve hours.
6. **Avoid alcohol close to bedtime.** Although a nightcap may make you feel sleepy, alcohol can disrupt sleep by causing nighttime awakenings.

you. If you notice that you wake up to use the bathroom in the middle of the night and can't fall back asleep, try cutting back on fluids late in the day.

According to some studies, exercising too close to bedtime can make falling asleep more difficult if your body doesn't have a chance to cool down. But that probably applies only to people who do very vigorous, sweaty workouts. If exercising in the evening works best for your schedule and doesn't seem to affect your sleep, there's no reason to change that habit.

In my experience, both personally and for my patients, sleep troubles are far more likely to stem from a mental rather than a physical cause. By mental, I mean stress or worry that keeps your mind racing and hard to settle. Both regular exercise and the relaxation techniques described in the next chapter go a long way toward solving this common problem. Waking up at night does not necessarily mean you cannot fall back asleep and feel refreshed in the morning, particularly if you have budgeted seven or more hours for sleep.

OTHER SUGGESTIONS FOR TREATING SLEEP SHORTFALLS

What if you've tried the shut-eye solutions but still can't seem to get enough sleep on a regular basis? Because sleep is so important for reaching your new silhouette, finding the right treatment is key.

When to See a Doctor

More than 40 million Americans suffer from sleep disorders. Many aren't diagnosed, even though they're relatively easy to treat. Insomnia, the inability to fall sleep or to stay asleep throughout the night, is the most common sleep disorder. It may be a symptom of an underlying medical or psychological condition. If you have persistent problems getting enough sleep and often feel drowsy during the day, see your health care provider for an evaluation.

Sleep apnea, a common sleep disorder characterized by brief interruptions of breathing during sleep, affects an estimated 18 million Americans. The most common form of this problem, obstructive sleep apnea, occurs when something—the tongue, tonsils, or uvula (the little piece of flesh hanging in the back of the throat)—blocks the windpipe.

Overweight people are more prone to this problem, in part because excess fatty tissue in the throat can block the windpipe.

People who snore loudly and who have high blood pressure are more likely to have sleep apnea. If your bedmate complains about your loud snoring, that's a clear warning signal and should prompt a call to your physician. Sleep apnea doesn't just disrupt sleep but also raises the risk of heart disease.

Natural Sleep Aids

According to a survey from the National Center of Complementary and Alternative Medicine, 1.6 million Americans use nontraditional treatments to help them sleep, such as herbs (lavender and chamomile, for example) or the hormone melatonin. However, these therapies aren't very effective. And as with other supplements, you can't be sure what you're actually getting. Mind–body techniques, such as deep breathing exercises and meditation (detailed in the next chapter), may be more useful and are risk-free.

Over-the-Counter Sleep Aids

If you have trouble sleeping once in a while, an over-the-counter sleeping pill may be a good option. All contain the same active ingredient: an antihistamine. Commonly used to treat allergies, these drugs often cause drowsiness as a side effect, which is why they're used in sleeping pills. But don't use them for longer than a week or so, because people can develop tolerance to them after just four days. (Tolerance means your body no longer responds to the normal dose and requires higher doses to achieve the same effects.) Antihistamines can cause a morning "hangover" and many other side effects, including nausea, dizziness, and coordination problems. For these reasons, experts say that prescription medications are actually a better choice for chronic insomnia because they have fewer drawbacks.

Prescription Sleeping Pills

These medications fall into four general categories:

Melatonin receptor agonists: This new class of medication includes only one drug so far, called ramelteon (Rozerem), which works by attaching to the same brain receptors for melatonin produced naturally by the body. Its sleep-inducing effects are more potent that over-the-counter melatonin supplements.

Nonbenzodiazepine hypnotics: This category of drugs works by quieting the nervous system. Because they break down quickly in the body, next-day side effects are relatively uncommon. They include zolpidem (Ambien), zaleplon (Sonata), and eszopiclone (Lunesta).

Benzodiazepine hypnotics: These older sleeping pills are more likely to cause side effects such as drowsiness or headaches the following day, compared with the newer pills. They include triazolam (Halcion), estazolam (Prosom), and temazepam (Restoril).

Antidepressants: Some older antidepressant drugs also cause drowsiness at low doses and may be helpful for people whose sleep problems are secondary to depression or anxiety. They include trazodone (Desyrel), amitriptyline (Amitril, Elavil), and nortriptyline (Aventyl, Pamelor).

All these medications have side effects and should be used no longer than a few weeks to address a short-term problem. If you have chronic insomnia, work with a specialist to get to the root of the problem rather than simply treating the symptoms. Insomnia is often undertreated—but drugs are overused and often prescribed for long-term use on a regular basis, even though they're intended to be for short-term intermittent use.

Transitioning to More Sleep

As with the other steps of the set point solution, make changes slowly to reach a target of seven to eight hours of sleep per night. If you normally go to bed around 11:30, try going to bed fifteen minutes earlier for a week. Once you've adjusted to that new time, move it back another fifteen minutes, continuing that pattern until you reach a schedule that leaves you feeling energized and ready to go when you awaken. It will take time—at least several weeks, if not longer—to achieve this goal. As you're mastering sleep, start looking at your time budget.

WHERE DOES YOUR TIME GO?

To get a sense of where you spend your time, start with a balance of twenty-four hours. Tailor the table to fit your day by subtracting the amount of time you sleep, work, commute, eat and prepare food, exercise, tend to family members, perform housework, watch TV, work or play on the computer, read, shop, and so on. See what time is left in the day and if there are unnecessary activities you can cut. Ideally, your weekend time management accounting table will afford you plenty of extra time to catch up on physical activity, leisure time, family time, errands, house and yard work, and preparation for the week so that weekdays are somewhat more manageable. Try to avoid the temptation of taking extra or longer naps to make up for staying up too late.

Of course, this scenario is a little too simple. We all have different responsibilities that don't fit into those neat time allocations. For example, many people spend additional time caring for small children or elderly relatives. And time challenges and constraints vary from day to day; for example, if you need to get your car repaired or your teeth cleaned. Still, if you take a hard look at how you spend the hours that you're not sleeping, working, or doing other necessary chores, you may find that you have more free time than you realize. For many people,

SAMPLE WEEKDAY TIME MANAGEMENT
ACCOUNTING TABLE

24 hours −8 hours	**Total** (on average, for sleep)
16 hours −1 hour	**Remaining** (getting ready in morning: stretching or other exercise, showering, breakfast, getting kids ready, reading newspaper)
15 hours −1 hour	**Remaining** (commuting, transporting children and family, potential recreational time or a physically active commute)
14 hours −8.5 hours	**Remaining** (8-hour workday +30-minute lunch break, or a combination of work with child care and errands, housework)
5.5 hours −1 hour	**Remaining** (commuting, transporting children and family, after-school activities/ sports, potential recreational time or a physically active commute)
4.5 hours −2 hours	**Remaining** (for meal preparation, dinner, cleaning up, packing next day's lunch, miscellaneous chores)

2.5 hours	**Remaining**
	(for physical activity, exercise, family/leisure time—helping the
	    kids with their homework, playing games, reading, exploring, maybe
	    watching an hour of TV, getting ready for tomorrow, relaxing, catching
	    up with family/friends on the phone)

watching television makes up a large part of their leisure time. Time spent using other forms of media—especially computers—is another growing trend in our society.

Computer Conundrum

Sometimes, using computers may actually save time; for example, when people use them to do online shopping or to pay bills. But the most common computer-related pursuits include Web surfing, emailing, instant messaging, and playing online games. According to a study from the Stanford Institute for the Quantitative Study of Society, surfing the Web and playing games were the most commonly reported activities on the Internet. The study also found that people who use the Internet are more likely to sleep less. However, researchers found that time spent on the Internet mainly takes away from discretionary time, like social activities, hobbies, and reading, and has less of an impact on time spent on mandatory activities such as work and sleep. In any case, it's worth keeping track of how much time you spend on your computer and experimenting with ways to make your screen time more efficient, such as checking your personal email only once or twice a day instead of numerous times. I also recommend carving out a tech-free time during the weekend for at least four hours. Unplug yourself from your computer, cell phone, Blackberry, and related devices and spend the time relaxing, exercising, or socializing with family and friends.

The Trouble with TV

Americans watch an average of four hours and thirty-two minutes of television every day. Watching TV has been linked to excess weight in both children and adults. Still, television is a prominent part of many people's daily lives, and there's no reason to cut it out completely. But if you watch more than three hours each day, consider cutting back to just one to two hours per day, selecting just a few programs you really enjoy. If they're on at 10:00 or 11:00 P.M., record them to watch another night at 9:00. Taming your TV habit is probably the simplest way to build in extra time for exercising and preparing healthy meals. Another trick is multitasking: doing something else productive while you watch TV. Just make sure the other activity is productive, not destructive.

Good

Exercising: You can just do some simple stretches, sit-ups, or leg lifts on the carpet, or set up a treadmill or stationary bike in front of the TV.

Doing chores. Try folding laundry, mending, or doing other tasks you can do on your lap. You can also make to-do lists or update your address book or day planner during the commercial breaks. If you have a TV in your kitchen, watch while you cook or clean up.

Bad

Lying down while you watch TV: This burns even fewer calories than sitting! Remember my NEAT tips from Chapter 7.

Watching late-night shows: Chances are that watching these programs is keeping you up too late.

Ugly

Eating: This is bad news for several reasons. First, eating while you're engaged in any another activity—even one as passive as television watching—isn't a good idea. You can become easily distracted and eat more than you intend to: the classic mindless eating syndrome. Second, eating just before you go to bed (when most people tend to watch TV) isn't good for your digestion. Food that is not properly digested can lead to heartburn and disrupted sleep. In addition to mindless eating syndrome, people tend to eat calorie-laden snacks at night in front of the TV, such as chips, cookies, ice cream, and popcorn.

PLANNING YOUR ROUTINE

Jot down a schedule for a typical weekday in your journal. You can also use you Palm Pilot or Day Planner, or copy the blank forms in the Appendix. Remember that your sleep time is your most important priority.

Writing these tasks down will help you stay organized. As I mentioned before, your weekend days can be used to complete tasks that are tricky to squeeze in during the week.

SAMPLE WEEKDAY SCHEDULE

Time	To Do	Hours
6:00 A.M.	Rise, stretch, watch news and walk on treadmill for 30 minutes	1 hour
7:00 A.M.	Eat breakfast with husband, shower, prepare for work	1 hour
8:00 A.M.	Commute to work	30 minutes
8:30 A.M.	Work	3½ hours
12:00 P.M.	Brisk walk during lunch break	30 minutes
12:30 P.M.	Work	5 hours
5:30 P.M.	Commute home	30 minutes
6:00 P.M.	Take dog for a walk to town center, pick up extra groceries	1 hour
7:00 P.M.	Prepare and eat dinner with family, pack up leftovers for lunch tomorrow	1 hour
8:00 P.M.	Watch evening news, vacuum during commercial breaks	1 hour
9:00 P.M.	Lay out clothes for tomorrow, read, make to-do list	1 hour
10:00 P.M.	Nighttime routine and into bed	8 hours

SAMPLE SUNDAY SCHEDULE

Time	To Do	Hours
7:00 AM	Rise, stretch, eat breakfast, and read the paper	2 hours
9:00 AM	Brisk walk around the neighborhood with the dog	1 hour
10:00 AM	Plan out week's meals, make a list	1 hour
11:00 AM	Go grocery shopping	1 hour
12:00 PM	Precut vegetables for the week, bag up nuts and crackers for snacks	1 hour

Time	To Do	Hours
1:00 PM	Tech-free time: No TV or computer until this evening! Go for a hike with a friend, take a group exercise class, or take the kids to a museum	4 hours
5:00 PM	Prepare and eat dinner with family, pack up leftovers for lunch tomorrow	2 hours
7:00 PM	Catch up on email and phone calls, do laundry	2 hours
9:00 PM	Lay out clothes for tomorrow, read, make to-do list	1 hour
10:00 PM	Nighttime routine and into bed	9 hours

One of the best things about going to bed early is that it allows you to wake up earlier, giving you extra time in the morning to focus on yourself. I find that having an hour in the morning to exercise, read the paper, and enjoy my breakfast at a leisurely pace really helps set the stage for a productive, positive day. All too often, people rush around in the morning, trying to organize themselves (and their families) for the entire day. Give yourself a break and plan ahead the night before: make your lunch, lay out your clothes, jot down your to-do list before you go to bed. Knowing you're already set for the next day can help you relax and go to sleep.

Don't forget to factor in some flexibility. For instance, say you planned to get up early to take a walk before work but you overslept. Instead, make up the exercise time by riding a stationary bike while you watch television at night, or exercise for twice as long on the next weekend day.

Enlist the help of your family and friends, which can boost the chances of sticking with the plan. If you agree to meet a friend to exercise together at a specific time, you're more likely to show up. Ask your spouse or partner to pitch in with some of the food shopping, such as picking up fresh fruits and vegetables midweek so that you don't have to make that extra trip to the store. Help one another resist those late evening TV shows and get to bed earlier.

EXERCISE TIME-SAVERS

Add Exercise to Your Commute

- Walk (or if possible, bike) all or part of your route to work.

- Get on or off the bus/subway/train one or two stops before your destination.

- If you drive, park at the farthest spot away in the lot.

- Take the stairs instead of the elevator; if you can't manage walking up all the flights, start with just one or two flights and build up.

Exercise at Work

- Take a walk outside, or in a nearby mall if the weather's bad.

- Join a fitness club or pool near your workplace.

- Ask your human resources department about the possibility of company-sponsored exercise classes at your workplace, held before, during, or after work.

- If you need to communicate with a colleague, walk to his or her office instead of picking up the phone or sending an email.

- If appropriate, swap your office chair for a stability ball (see the Appendix) and put all of those small, stabilizing muscles to work during the day.

Exercise at Home

- Buy an exercise video or treadmill/stationary bike so that you can exercise at home on your own schedule. This saves the time spent driving to and from a gym or health club.

- Small, inexpensive gadgets like resistance bands and hand weights can supplement exercise videos and home exercises.

- Incorporate exercise into your leisure time.

- Instead of meeting friends for coffee or cocktails, take a walk or hike while you visit.

- Find a fun exercise you can do with your family or friends: hiking, biking, in-line skating, cross-country skiing.

- Do your own gardening and yard work.

Food-Related Ways to Save Time

- Plan general menus in advance, use and make a shopping list, and go to the store only once or twice weekly.

- Consider using a grocery delivery service, which saves time driving to the store and shopping.

- Buy precut vegetables and fruits.

- Use frozen and canned foods, particularly fruits and vegetables.

- Prepare enough food so that leftovers can be incorporated into the next day's meal.

- Assemble tomorrow's lunch while you make tonight's dinner and save on cleanup time.

- Take advantage of the grocery store salad bar to supplement a homemade salad.

- See the Appendix for quick weeknight recipes.

Do not eat while walking, traveling, using the computer, or watching TV. Eating on the run won't allow you to spend the vital twenty minutes you need to feel full. You may think you're saving time by grabbing coffee and a muffin on the way to work instead of pouring yourself a bowl of cereal, but are you considering the detour (however minor) and the additional time to park and stand in line? Also, don't skip a meal in order to make more time for errands or chores.

Multitask While You Exercise

- Read or watch the news.
- Read a magazine or book, or do a crossword puzzle.
- Spend quality time with your spouse, kids, or friends.
- Walk around the soccer field while you watch your kids play sports.
- Conduct a business or neighborhood meeting on foot.
- Use vigorous house cleaning as a way to exercise.
- Walk around the block while you catch up with friends on your cell phone.

NINE

Stress-Fighting Solutions and the Happiness Factor

Pleasure is the good feeling that comes from satisfying homeostatic needs such as hunger, sex, and bodily comfort. Enjoyment, on the other hand, refers to the good feeling people experience when they break through the limits of homeostasis—when they do something that stretches them beyond what they were—in an athletic event, an artistic performance, a good deed, a stimulating conversation. Enjoyment, rather than pleasure, is what leads to personal growth and long-term happiness, but why is that when given a chance, most people opt for pleasure over enjoyment?

—Martin E. P. Seligman, Ph.D.,
professor of psychology,
University of Pennsylvania, and
Mihaly Csikszentmihalyi, Ph.D.,
professor of psychology,
Claremont Graduate University

MATT'S STORY: DEALING WITH WORK-RELATED STRESS

When Matt, a 50-year-old accountant, first came to us, he routinely skipped breakfast, overate at lunch, and couldn't find time to exercise. We helped him make small, gradual changes to reset his set point. He began waking up twenty minutes earlier so that he could eat breakfast and cut back on his fast-food runs. Matt joined a gym so that he could start working out three to four times a week after work. After four months, he said he never felt better, and his new habits were becoming second nature.

Then, tax season rolled around. The added workload prompted him to quit going to the gym. His overall energy level started to dip, and he began hitting the snooze button on his alarm instead of getting up to eat breakfast. He sensed his stress level rising, not just because of the extra work, but also because he felt discouraged and guilty about how easily he slid back into his old habits. Matt wondered if getting back on track would even be worth the effort. Given how easily he'd abandoned his routine, what would prevent him from doing the same thing in the future?

Luckily, he checked in with us before throwing in the towel. We encouraged him to look at his situation not as a setback but as a learning experience that would strengthen his skills in finding flexible solutions during future times of stress. We also advised him to mark a date on the calendar when his routine would likely return to normal so that he could see the changes were temporary. In the meantime, we looked at his original plan to see how we could tweak it. He had been eating oatmeal for breakfast, but we agreed that he could switch to meal replacements or bars a few times a week to save time. He also decided to make hard-boiled eggs on Sundays so that he could bring them to work for a snack or as part of a meal.

Going to the gym during or after work wasn't realistic, since he often saw clients all day long and sometimes into the evening. We suggested that Matt try to get unstructured short bursts of activity during the week and go to the gym on the weekend. He began parking farther away from his office, taking the stairs, and walking around his building between clients. He didn't think he'd find time to meditate for ten minutes during the day, but he added some deep breathing exercises to help him relax when work became especially tense.

Together, we mapped out a busy season plan that still touched upon Matt's original goals but in a more flexible manner. Matt realized that in the coming years, he would have less stress at tax time because he had a plan ready to go.

SARAH'S STORY: COPING WHEN A FAMILY MEMBER BECOMES SERIOUSLY ILL

Sarah, age 47, had been progressing well with the set point program. A mother of two who worked full-time as a nurse, she had made major improvements in her eating habits, by cutting back on high-fat treats, cooking healthier meals, and bringing her lunch to work. She'd also begun to exercise regularly. Then Sarah's mother, a cancer survivor, was hospitalized with a relapse. Sarah often went to the hospital after work to visit her mother, so she wasn't able to cook dinner. Exhausted and emotionally drained after these visits, she would either stop by the hospital cafeteria for a cookie or the drive-through doughnut place on her way home. She was waking up in the middle of the night, worrying about her mother, and she often ended up in the kitchen looking for something to nibble on.

Sarah felt out of control and was afraid that this feeling would trickle down and dismantle the entire healthy lifestyle plan she had worked so hard to develop. We suggested that she identify for herself the things that she could control. She realized that while she couldn't stop worrying about her mother, she still had control over what she ate and how much activity she did. But she felt so down in the dumps that she was afraid she couldn't muster the effort to make healthy choices. We recommended simplifying her current plan and then committing it to paper. We decided she would have a meal replacement or frozen entree for lunch to cut down on her shopping and preparation time. She also asked for support and delegated dinner responsibilities to other family members three nights a week. Both of these changes left her more time and eased her stress a bit.

We discussed recognizing the difference between eating when you're hungry and eating when you're upset or sad (emotional eating). We suggested some strategies to help her avoid the cafeteria or doughnut shop. For example, she could keep a portion-controlled sweet treat (such as a 100-calorie snack pack of cookies or even a miniature chocolate bar) in her purse or car. Sarah came up with different activities she could do when she woke up at night, such as knitting, reading, or listening to a meditation CD. With these suggestions and the support of her family, she managed to keep on track and maintain her weight during that difficult period.

DAILY STRESS

Once you master the prescriptions detailed in Chapters 5 through 8, you will look and feel better. Thanks to your new structured lifestyle, a lower weight, and higher fitness level, your overall stress level will likely drop a bit.

As in the cases of Matt and Sarah, the unavoidable stresses of everyday life can slow your progress toward reaching your new set point. A 2006 survey by the American Psychological Association (APA) found that nearly half of all Americans are concerned about the amount of stress in their lives, and many of them resort to unhealthy habits such as comfort eating as a means of coping. Also known as emotional eating, this habit is a common reaction not only to stress but to other negative emotions, such as anger, anxiety, boredom, sadness, and loneliness. The APA also reports that 43% of all adults suffer adverse health effects from stress and that at least 75% of all physician office visits are for stress-related ailments and complaints. That's no surprise when you consider that six of the leading causes of death—heart disease, cancer, lung ailments, accidents, cirrhosis of the liver, and suicide—are linked to stress.

Most diet books don't give enough attention to the mental aspects of weight loss and long-term weight control. Just as the internal factors in your body that control your weight strive toward balance, you also need balance in the external aspects of your life. These factors include how much you eat, exercise, and sleep, but also how much you work, play, and relax, which affects your emotional well-being. Staying balanced when life's problems start to feel overwhelming is hard. But a number of different strategies to quell stress and enhance happiness can help.

Medically speaking, stress is the body's normal physical response to anything that requires you to adjust to change. Stress triggers the fight or flight response, the ingrained survival mechanism that helps you react quickly in the face of danger, be it a wild animal or a car speeding toward you. We all know the immediate physical sensations of stress: the heart pounds, muscles tighten, breathing quickens, and sweating increases.

The stress response has positive effects even in everyday environments. Lesser threats, like an impending deadline, can boost your performance and efficiency. But after a certain point, stress can overwhelm you, causing a drop in productivity. And unfortunately, our bodies aren't good at telling the difference between life-threatening events and day-to-day stressful situations, such as an argument with a loved one or a bad traffic jam.

So-called stressors vary from minor inconveniences to major life traumas. Traumatic stressors include the death of a spouse or other close relative; divorce or separation; a major illness or injury; and getting fired from your job. People often develop physical symptoms in response to severe stress, such as headaches, stomachaches, and a loss of appetite. Coping with stress from these life-altering changes goes beyond the scope of this chapter and is often best addressed by working with a personal therapist.

The body's response to nontraumatic stressors, or daily annoyances and worries, is often more subtle. But the effects may be longer lasting and more problematic. Chronic stress may contribute to or exacerbate a wide range of health problems, including digestive woes such as heartburn and constipation, high blood pressure and heart problems, and pain (head or muscle aches, for example). Take some time to consider the sources of stress in your life, which can be from the outside world (external stressors) or from within you (internal stressors).

External Stress

- *Money:* Are you concerned about paying bills or saving for retirement? (Financial worries are also intimately linked to the next two stressors.)

- *Home and family:* Do you have frequent spats with your spouse, a child with behavior problems, or an elderly ill parent?

- *Work:* Are you coping with a heavy workload, an impatient boss, or difficult coworkers?

- *Environment:* Do you have a long, difficult commute to work? Is the neighbor's leaf blower or yapping dog driving you nuts? On a larger scale, you might be stressed about the state of the world, the country, or any local community to which you belong.

Internal Stress

Some of these stressors stem from bad habits, which are sometimes a reaction to other forms of stress. Others may just be part of who you are, based on your genes and the environment in which you grew up.

- *Irresponsible behavior:* Do you put yourself in risky or dangerous situations?

- *Poor health habits:* Do you smoke, drink excessively, or use illegal drugs?

- *Negative attitudes:* Do you often feel pessimistic, uncertain, or fearful?

- *Unrealistic expectations:* Do you have perfectionist tendencies or are you overly controlling?

To get a sense of your general stress level, take the stress test.

PERCEIVED STRESS SCALE

The questions in this scale ask you about your feelings and thoughts during the last month. In each case, please indicate with a check how often you felt or thought a certain way.

1. In the last month, how often have you been upset because of something that happened unexpectedly?
___0 = never ___1 = almost never ___2 = sometimes ___3 = fairly often ___4 = very often

2. In the last month, how often have you felt that you were unable to control the important things in your life?
___0 = never ___1 = almost never ___2 = sometimes ___3 = fairly often ___4 = very often

3. In the last month, how often have you felt nervous and stressed?
___0 = never ___1 = almost never ___2 = sometimes ___3 = fairly often ___4 = very often

4. In the last month, how often have you felt confident about your ability to handle your personal problems?
___0 = very often ___1 = fairly often ___2 = sometimes ___3 = almost never ___4 = never

5. In the last month, how often have you felt that things were going your way?
___0 = very often ___1 = fairly often ___2 = sometimes ___3 = almost never ___4 = never

6. In the last month, how often have you found that you could not cope with all the things that you had to do?
___0 = never ___1 = almost never ___2 = sometimes ___3 = fairly often ___4 = very often

7. In the last month, how often have you been able to control irritations in your life?
___0 = very often ___1 = fairly often ___2 = sometimes ___3 = almost never ___4 = never

8. In the last month, how often have you felt that you were on top of things?
___0 = very often ___1 = fairly often ___2 = sometimes ___3 = almost never ___4 = never

9. In the last month, how often have you been angered by things beyond your control?
___0 = never ___1 = almost never ___2 = sometimes ___3 = fairly often ___4 = very often

10. In the last month, how often have you felt difficulties were piling up so high that you could not overcome them?
___0 = never ___1 = almost never ___2 = sometimes ___3 = fairly often ___4 = very often

Scoring:

0–13 points
Low: A low stress level bodes well for your health and ability to maintain a weight-loss program. Keep practicing whatever stress management strategies you're using now. However, it's normal to fluctuate and experience periods of higher stress, so stay aware of your stress levels and continue to practice the stress management strategies that work best for you.

(continued)

PERCEIVED STRESS SCALE (*continued*)

14–27 points
Moderate: Moderate stress is completely normal, as long as it doesn't last for weeks or months on end. Over time, even lower levels of stress can affect your ability to maintain a healthy lifestyle. Start taking steps now to address your stress levels, by working to eliminate possible stressors and practicing relaxation techniques.

28–40 points
High: Being under a lot of stress—especially for an extended period of time—can damage your health, including your mental health and your immune system. Do whatever you can to eliminate some of those sources of stress and practice the stress management strategies that work best for you, whether that's exercising, unwinding with friends, or meditating. Consider asking your health care provider or friend for a referral to a therapist.

Source: Based on Dr. S. Cohen, Carnegie Mellon University, 10-Item Perceived Stress Scale, 1988.

COPING MECHANISMS

Unfortunately, some common ways people cope with stress can overturn their set point efforts. For example, watching television can be relaxing, but that depends on what (and when) you watch, as I've mentioned before. Poor sleep is both a cause and a symptom of stress. Likewise, drinking alcohol may ease tension, but too much can lead to disinhibition and overeating.

Finally, like Sarah, many people turn to food when they're stressed. Researchers have published studies in rats suggesting that cortisol plays a role in this phenomenon. A high level of this hormone, which is produced in response to stress, prompts animals to seek out high-energy foods (for the rats, sugar and lard). The resulting fat deposits, which are found mainly in the belly area, may send a signal that puts the brakes on the stress response. These findings give new meaning to the concept of comfort foods, which tend to be high in fat and sugar and may actually bring about a sense of calm.

As already noted, stress is only one of the emotions that triggers emotional eating. People may eat more when they're sad, unhappy, or distressed. A 2007 study found that people watching a sad movie (*Love Story,* a 1970s tear-jerker) gobbled down about 28% more popcorn than those watching a recent romantic comedy (*Sweet Home Alabama*). The same study also reported that college students who read news of a fire that killed seven children ate four times as many M&Ms as raisins from nearby bowls of snacks, whereas students who read about the chance reunion of four old friends ate more raisins than M&Ms. A brief "Eating Habits" quiz may help you tune in to your propensity for emotional eating.

EATING HABITS

Please indicate the degree to which you believe each of the following behaviors causes you to gain weight. In answering these questions, please use the 5-point scale below. Pick the one number that best describes how much behavior contributes to your increased weight.

1. does not contribute at all
2. contributes a small amount
3. contributes a moderate amount
4. contributes a large amount
5. contributes the greatest amount
__(a) eating with family/friends
__(b) eating when socializing/celebrating
__(c) eating at business functions
__(d) eating when happy
__(e) eating in response to sight or smell of food
__(f) eating because of the good taste of foods
__(g) eating because I can't stop once I've begun
__(h) overeating at dinner
__(i) eating too much food
__(j) continuing to eat because I don't feel full after a meal
__(k) eating because I crave certain foods
__(l) eating because I feel physically hungry
__(m) eating while cooking/preparing food
__(n) eating when stressed
__(o) eating when depressed/upset
__(p) eating when angry
__(q) eating when anxious
__(r) eating when alone
__(s) eating when bored
__(t) eating when tired
__(u) overeating at lunch
__(v) overeating at breakfast
__(w) snacking after dinner
__(x) snacking between meals

Source: Adapted from the "Weight and Lifestyle Inventory" by Gary Foster and Thomas Wadden.

POSITIVE WAYS TO HANDLE STRESS

For our purposes, the point of the "Eating Habits" quiz isn't to tally your score so much as to raise your awareness of whether you're eating out of physical hunger or psychological hunger (sometimes referred to as "stomach hunger" and "mouth hunger"). Most of the quiz items are situations in which you are feeding your mouth hunger. The bottom line is that if you follow the 450-calorie twenty-minute rule, you will reach a comfortable level of fullness. For the subsequent three to four hours, anything you eat will be fulfilling your mouth hunger, not your stomach hunger. But here's the deal: It's perfectly fine to feed your mouth hunger, as long as you keep the amount to a reasonable limit. If you control the portion size at all of your meals, you'll have an extra 100 to 200 discretionary calories. Go ahead and enjoy that small piece of chocolate or whatever you're craving. Other favorite comfort foods, like macaroni and cheese or mashed potatoes, are fine, too. Eat one serving slowly! You can also make healthier versions of traditional comfort foods (see the Appendix for Chapter 6).

Once you've identified the stressors in your life and how you respond to them, consider some alternative ways to manage stress. One tactic is to reduce stress-inducing circumstances. If your schedule is too busy, politely say no when people ask for your help with volunteer activities. If possible, change your schedule to avoid a bad commute. Avoid people or situations that aggravate you.

But most of the time, you will face events you can't control. Taking care of yourself physically, by following the set point strategies, can help a great deal—especially the prescription for exercise, which is a great stress reliever. You also need to nurture your mental health to stay in balance. To that end, I recommend mind–body techniques. Cognitive behavioral therapy can also be very helpful, both for relieving stress and enhancing weight loss.

Mind-Body Techniques

These techniques represent different ways to elicit the relaxation response, a concept championed and studied by Herbert Benson, M.D., an associate professor of medicine at Harvard Medical School and director emeritus of the Benson-Henry Institute for Mind Body Medicine. This response creates a feeling of deep rest that generates physical changes in the body mediated through the autonomic nervous system. In particular, these techniques help lower your body's "fight or flight" response and enhance the "rest and digest" response. You can practice these techniques during the day, in the evening, or even while in bed.

Progressive Muscle Relaxation: Isolating specific sets of muscles, tensing them briefly, and then relaxing them creates a sense of release and letting go that can quiet a racing mind. Start at the top of your head and move down to your toes.

Deep breathing: This technique is intended to mimic the deep, slow breathing that's typical during sleep, which stems from the diaphragm, the muscle between the abdomen and chest. While lying down:

1. Place one hand on your chest and one on your stomach.

2. Slowly inhale through your nose or through pursed lips (to slow the breath).

3. Feel your stomach expand, which should cause your hand to rise.

4. Slowly exhale through pursed lips.

5. Try to match the length of the exhale to the length of your inhale.

6. Rest and repeat five to ten times.

Meditation: This practice encourages you to focus your thoughts on the present moment, with a goal of quieting the mind's distractions, not thinking about the past or the future. You can take meditation classes, and most yoga classes include meditation as well. Or try it on your own:

1. Sit quietly in a comfortable position with your eyes closed.

2. Relax your muscles and take a deep, slow breath.

3. Choose a focus word or short phrase, perhaps one that resonates with your religious or spiritual beliefs (for example, "one," "peace," "amen," or "shalom").

4. As you breathe, repeat the word aloud or in your mind.

5. Assume a passive attitude, without concern about how well you're doing. When other thoughts come to mind, simply say to yourself, "Oh well," and gently return to your repetition.

6. Continue for ten to twenty minutes.

Visualization or Guided Imagery: A variant of meditation, this practice encourages you to focus on soothing images to help you relax. You can conjure up your own images—a scene, place, experience—or work with a therapist who verbalizes pleasant images, such as beaches or forests. You can also buy recordings that will help you practice this technique (see the Appendix).

Cognitive Behavioral Therapy

Cognitive behavioral therapy (CBT) is a short-term form of therapy that's widely used for a number of disorders, including anxiety, panic attacks, insomnia, and weight loss. Unlike other forms of talk therapy, CBT requires work on the patient's part. Therapists often assign homework to their patients, such as having them keep track of certain habits and practicing alternative ways of thinking that might make them feel better. Some studies suggest that people undergoing behavioral therapy lose between 8% and 10% of their weight in six months, and CBT is especially effective when used in tandem with diet and exercise strategies.

In essence, CBT provides an individualized and more focused approach to some of the things I've described in this and other chapters of the book. Unlike psychotherapy, which dwells on the origins of your problems, CBT focuses on the here and now. During the treatment, the therapist helps the patient discover and expose negative ways of thinking, irrational beliefs, and unhealthy habits, and suggests ways to replace them with more positive thoughts and behaviors. Negative thoughts often spur negative behaviors, as in Matt's case, when stress and guilt led him into a downward spiral. It's a common scenario among dieters: once they've blown their diet, they feel disgusted and upset, which can create a vicious cycle of overeating and a return to unhealthy habits.

In CBT directed toward weight loss, the therapist helps the patient set realistic goals for weight loss and behavior changes. Patients also learn to gauge their success in modifying their eating and activity habits and to correct negative thoughts that crop up when they experience slips. A key tenet of the therapy is setting specific goals that can be readily achieved and easily measured. For example, you might set a goal to walk four times a week, lengthen your evening meal by ten minutes, and cut down on the number of self-critical comments you make over the course of a day. Next, you might consider things that can either help or hinder your ability to reach those goals. Rather than making drastic, unsustainable, and unrealistic changes, you learn to make small, gradual changes and build on your success over time.

Give Yourself a Break: Understanding Behavior Chains

Therapists use various tools to facilitate cognitive and behavioral changes. One helpful tool is a behavior chain, which refers to a series of sometimes minor events that lead to an undesirable outcome, like overeating. By looking back at what occurred before you overate, you can re-create you own behavior chain. For example, maybe you tossed and turned the previous night, so you overslept and skipped breakfast. By lunchtime, you were ravenous and wolfed down a fast-food meal. Afterward, you felt guilty, but by late afternoon you were hungry again. Your boss stopped by to say she needed something urgent done before you left work, so you went to the candy machine for a snack. In this example, you can probably identify several places where you could have broken the chain. For instance, you could have practiced a relaxation technique to help you sleep better. Also, you could have stocked up on healthy snacks to keep at your desk.

The earlier you break the chain, the better. It takes practice to realize how small, seemingly unimportant thoughts or behaviors early in a chain may lead to uncontrolled eating or poor food choices. Remember

SAMPLE BEHAVIOR CHAIN

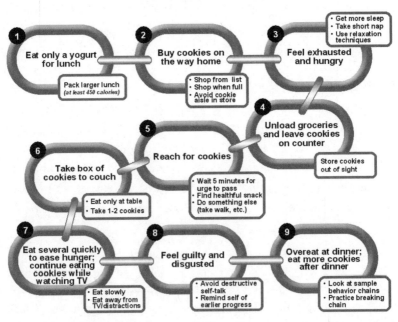

This sample behavior chain includes suggestions for breaking the links.

to ask for help from people around you. Find a family member to hide the cookies so that you can't break into them. If your behavior chain leads you to skip exercise after your walking partner cancels, ask your daughter or husband to take a walk with you instead. Remember that it takes time and practice to make these changes, so give yourself a break when learning them.

Finally, I want to stress that CBT isn't something you can learn from a book. You need a therapist to realize the full benefits. Most weight-loss programs affiliated with hospitals or other institutions in major cities offer CBT, both for individuals and groups.

CULTIVATING HAPPINESS

As you work on banishing negative thoughts and behaviors, you might find inspiration from the burgeoning field of positive psychology. Instead of focusing solely on the negative aspects of mental health, such as depression, anxiety, and neurosis, psychologists have begun embracing the other side of the coin by asking: What makes people happy?

The father of the field, Martin Seligman, Ph.D., describes three distinct routes to happiness: (1) having positive feelings, (2) being actively engaged in your life, and (3) having a sense of purpose or meaning outside of yourself. Interestingly, he and other experts have described a happiness set point, which is similar to a body-weight set point. Your overall level of satisfaction may rest partly in your genes, and no matter what happens in your life—good, bad, magnificent, or dreadful—you will probably settle back to your set range. But just as you can change your weight set point, you can also change your happiness set point.

Keys to Happiness

Regardless of your circumstances, you can make positive changes that will boost your happiness. If you've been following my set point weight-loss plan, you're already on your way. Throughout this book, I've made a conscious effort to focus on the positive, by telling you what you can do, not what you can't. Two of the practical suggestions positive psychologists recommend for achieving a more satisfying life focus on the same things I encourage:

1. Take care of your physical health.

2. Find good ways to cope with stress.

As they say, good health is a major source of wealth; without it, happiness is almost impossible. You may be surprised to learn that having lots of money doesn't guarantee happiness. Researchers have found that once your basic needs are met, a higher salary does little to boost your happiness quotient. Neither does being smart or having a good education. According to Seligman's research, strengths of the heart, such as zest, gratitude, hope, and love, are what bring people joy. How can you tap into those feelings? Here are some suggestions from positive psychology experts:

Make connections. In his book *Connect,* Edward Hallowell, M.D., who directs the Hallowell Center for Cognitive and Emotional Health in Sudbury, Massachusetts, wrote, "If I have seen one change make people feel better most often, it is finding a meaningful connection—to a person, to a job, to a club or team, to an institution, to God." Cultivate relationships by spending quality time with family members, a partner, friends, even pets. Make a conscious effort to gather for family suppers, meet friends for coffee, walk with a neighbor, or catch up with long-distance family and friends over the phone.

Count your blessings. Too often, we take our lives for granted. Take a moment to think about the things you appreciate about your life. Sonja Lyubomirsky, Ph.D., a professor of psychology at the University of California, Riverside, found that regularly writing down three to five things for which you feel thankful (a gratitude journal) can boost happiness.

Practice kindness. Make an effort to be kind and helpful, both to friends and strangers, by doing small favors they'll appreciate, like raking your neighbor's lawn or letting someone take a parking space you wanted. Doing good makes you feel good, so find ways to give back, by being a good friend and neighbor, acting as a mentor or big brother or big sister to someone, or doing volunteer or charity work.

Be more mindful. Staying focused in the present moment and taking time to notice new things (the practice of mindfulness, which I introduced in Chapter 5 with respect to eating) can foster happiness. Take time to appreciate sensual pleasures and wonders, like the smell of a pine forest or the taste of a mango. Create visually pleasing scenes, even in simple ways, like using nice placemats and candles with dinner, which my wife and I do regularly. Some psychologists recommend taking mental photographs of pleasurable moments to share with others or recall later when you're feeling blue.

TEN

Making the Set Point Solution Work for You

The problem is the mindset of Americans. They aren't willing to take a long-term approach. They want to go out and do it all at once, and despite decades of failure with that approach, that's still the way we approach weight management.

—James O. Hill, Ph.D.,
    professor of pediatrics and medicine,
    University of Colorado Health Sciences Center

If you want to keep lost pounds off, daily weighing is critical. But stepping on the scale isn't enough. You have to use that information to change your behavior, whether that means eating less or walking more. Paying attention to weight—and taking quick action if it creeps up— seems to be the secret to success.

—Rena Wing, Ph.D.,
    professor of psychiatry and human behavior,
    Brown Medical School

This final chapter begins with a profile of Carolyn, a woman I met while working on a project for a major northeastern supermarket chain designed to help shoppers identify healthful foods. Carolyn, who was project manager for the new program, mentioned that she'd decided to try to lose weight, spurred in part by the new knowledge she'd acquired about choosing healthy foods. But she went far beyond changing what she ate—she restructured her entire lifestyle. You'll see how the changes she made resonate well with the set point solution.

CAROLYN'S STORY: PUTTING IT ALL TOGETHER

A single mother who worked full-time, Carolyn had a history of yo-yo dieting. She'd tried low-fat and low-carb diets, as well as Weight Watchers. But the weight she lost always came back. While working on her company's campaign to help shoppers chose healthy foods, she was inspired to try again.

In addition to switching to whole-grain bread, she and her son started eating more fruit. Tricks such as putting a peeled orange in a baggie in the fridge and having an apple corer handy helped. Carolyn also started keeping healthy snacks, like a small baggie of almonds or low-fat string cheese, in her car and purse. She took advantage of her store's grocery delivery service, which saved her the time and hassle of driving to and from the store, not to mention coping with the crowds and lines. Instead of adding ice cream or other sweets to her grocery order, she began treating herself to a bouquet of fresh flowers.

Carolyn saved money on her food budget by cutting back on restaurant meals and built a repertoire of healthful, easy-to-prepare dinners. For example, she used her slow cooker to make soups or chili. Other favorites are bagged salad greens with precooked chicken strips and grilled whole-wheat pizza with black beans, corn, and barbecue sauce.

Writing down what and when she ate helped her realize her habit of late-night snacking, a relic from a childhood habit of eating Ding-Dongs while watching Johnny Carson. Going to bed earlier curbed that problem and helped her make her 5:00 A.M. meetings with her personal trainer. She joined a local gym after realizing she was eligible for a corporate membership. Carolyn does strength training, spinning, and takes a Jazzercise class. She uses a free online diet journal, www.fitday.com, to track her food, exercise, and weight-loss goals.

Carolyn feels that paying a personal trainer is a good investment, noting that she eventually progressed to meeting with the trainer just once every five weeks to get a new routine and track her progress. She treats these meetings and her exercise classes like doctor's appointments, because she considers them vital to her health. Carolyn's mother has high blood pressure and diabetes, and Carolyn was worried that if she didn't lose weight, she might end up with similar problems. She's also proud to be setting a good example for her 17-year-old son.

Carolyn decided to stop drinking for a while to see how that would affect the success of her diet. But when she went out with her friends, they'd sometimes give her a hard time. Carolyn grew up in a family whose ideal vacation was lying by a pool. Her newfound energy (thanks to extra sleep and her new exercise routine) spurred her to find new friends who enjoyed being active and healthy. She now drinks only occasionally, mindful of the calories in alcoholic beverages.

Carolyn lost 35 pounds over an eight-month period, a gradual loss that she should have no trouble maintaining. And her cholesterol level dropped from 273 to 200. For her, the time and effort was more than worthwhile in terms of the positive changes in her appearance and how she feels.

I'm betting that at least some of Carolyn's story sounds familiar to you. Like many people, she juggles her career and family and has a history of trying different diets. Her tipping point was two-fold: she learned more about healthful foods, and she recognized the possible health consequences of staying overweight by witnessing her mother's medical problems. Once she sought out more knowledge and support— from her trainer, to a large extent—she made it a priority to carry out her extreme makeover.

This book provides all the information and tools you need to do the same thing. Now, it's up to you to use this knowledge and make resetting your set point a priority in your life. One theme I've stressed several times is the need to individualize—to find what works best for *you*. You might find Carolyn's exercise routine inspiring and follow her lead, or you might want to do something completely different. After reading the different profiles in this book, I hope you'll borrow tips from one or more of them to create your own makeover.

And you don't even necessarily need to lose as much weight as Carolyn did. Many people have said to me, "I originally wanted to lose

50 pounds. But after I lost just 15 pounds, I realized that just a small amount of weight loss made a difference in how I looked and felt!" People come in all sizes. Not everyone can be a size 6, nor should they be. What's important is that you move toward a healthy weight for *you*, one silhouette at a time.

SILHOUETTES REVISITED

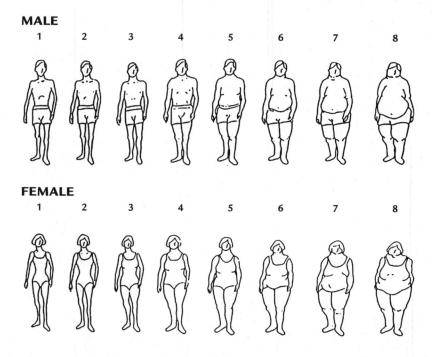

MALE
1   2   3   4   5   6   7   8

FEMALE
1   2   3   4   5   6   7   8

As Carolyn notes, putting all the pieces together really did the trick for her. Not only did she start eating less, eating well, and exercising, she retooled her schedule to make time for exercise and getting plenty of sleep. She built a new support network by cultivating new relationships. Carolyn "stretched her rubber band" but didn't let it snap—and went down two silhouettes (from silhouette 4 to silhouette 2) in less than one year.

STAYING THE COURSE: WHAT DOES IT TAKE?

One year into her weight-loss journey, Carolyn had managed to maintain her weight during the holiday season, despite being tempted by goodies at parties and a busier-than-normal schedule. She reset her set point and held her weight steady for a short time. As I explained in Chapter 3, holding steady once you reach a plateau will give your body time to readjust to your new set point.

Once you've reset your set point, the most challenging part of your journey is over. You've transformed and reorganized your daily routine to include more sleep, exercise, and satisfaction but with less food (especially junk food) and less stress. Sticking with these changes will allow you to stay the course. When you've mastered these new habits, your new lifestyle can last a lifetime.

But some people find that keeping weight off can be more difficult than taking it off. Part of it is just basic metabolism: Your body doesn't need as many calories to sustain your lower weight. And even when you lose weight gradually, you can't escape the fact that your body has become more fuel-efficient. One of the main reasons people regain weight is that they think only the initial weight-loss phase requires discipline, structure, and planning. Not true! That's why it's so important to select an eating and activity plan that is fun, realistic, and sustainable for the rest of your life.

Crash or fad diets inevitably fail because sticking to those regimens over the long term is not physically possible. We've all seen plenty of photos depicting slender people holding up their old oversized pants to document their amazing weight loss. I don't doubt that some of these are real people who actually have lost large amounts of weight. But these people are the exception, not the rule. Look at the fine print on the diet program ads, many of which say: "Results not typical." And I wonder what these atypical people look like after a year or two.

LESSONS FROM REAL LOSERS

Drs. Jim Hill and Rena Wing established the National Weight Control Registry (NWCR) in 1994. The registry is the largest prospective investigation of long-term successful weight-loss maintenance. Conventional wisdom says that people rarely succeed at long-term weight loss. But random digit dialing surveys suggest that about 20% of people in the general population report they have lost at least 10% of their weight and have kept it off for at least a year. To get a better handle on the keys to this success, the NWCR is tracking more than four thousand people who have successfully kept off 30 pounds or more for at least one year. Here are some facts about the registrants:

- Participants report having lost an average of 73 pounds and have kept that weight off for an average of 5.7 years.

- About half said they were overweight as children and 75% had at least one obese parent.

- Most (77%) are women, and the average age at joining the NWCR is 46.8 years.

- Nearly all have a history of trying to lose weight in the past, using numerous popular diet programs.

- About half lost weight on their own without any type of formal program or help.

- Most used both diet and physical activity to lose weight. Only 10% used diet alone and 1% used exercise alone.

An analysis of registry participants revealed six key strategies for keeping off lost weight over the long term:

1. Doing lots of physical activity: They exercise about sixty minutes daily, burning an average of 400 calories per session. Walking is the most frequently cited physical activity, listed by 77% of registrants. Women burn an average of 2,545 calories and men burn 3,293 calories weekly, which is equivalent to walking 20 to 30 miles per week. And one in five engage in weight training.

2. Eating a diet that's low in calories and fat: Registrants make an effort to eat few calories; in particular, they eat less fat and more fiber. On average, their diets hover around 24% fat, which is lower than the typical American diet.

3. Eating breakfast: Seventy-eight percent say they have breakfast every day. Their typical choice is my own favorite: cereal and fruit!

4. Weighing themselves regularly: Seventy-seven percent weigh themselves at least once a week and 44% weigh themselves daily.

5. Having consistent eating habits: Most say they follow the same eating patterns on weekdays and weekends, as well as during vacations and holidays. They eat at fast-food restaurants once a week and eat 2.5 meals per week at other restaurants, on average.

6. Catching slips before they turn into larger regains: Their frequent weight monitoring helps, but taking action is what really counts. Most participants keep close tabs on how much they eat, particularly if they gain more than a few pounds.

The study also notes that 83% of the participants reported a triggering event that spurred them to lose weight. Medical triggers, such as a doctor telling the participant to lose weight, or a family member having a heart attack or other serious medical problem, were the most common triggers. Reaching an all-time high in weight and seeing a picture or reflection of themselves in the mirror were other cited reasons.

Registry data reveal that successful losers tend to have fairly high dietary restraint scores (see Chapter 5). There's a fine line between being too rigid and too flexible when dieting, however. People who tended to be too flexible with their eating habits on holidays and vacations were more prone to regain weight, probably because they allowed themselves to disinhibit and overeat. Ideally, you should stick with your structured plan even when you're on vacation. But if you do overeat and underexercise away from home, the important thing is to get back to your healthy, structured schedule when you return. People who had fewer problems with disinhibition were more likely to keep off their lost weight over a year. Likewise, people who were less depressed tended to be more successful in maintaining weight loss, which supports the importance of emotional health, as described in Chapter 9.

Finally, here's some encouraging news: the longer you maintain your weight loss, the easier it is to keep it off. People in the registry who kept off lost pounds for two years or more were far more likely to maintain their weight over the following year. Also, among the people who did regain some of their lost weight, nearly all of them stayed more than 10% below their highest-ever weight. They dropped at least one set point—and that ranks as a victory in my book (and is also considered successful by current obesity treatment standards).

THE COSTS OF LOSING—AND NOT LOSING—WEIGHT

One of the biggest obstacles people face when they try to lose weight is believing that they can't afford to lose weight; namely, that eating healthful foods and exercising is too costly. The simple truth is that you can't afford to stay overweight.

Losing weight can be expensive if you throw your money away on useless weight-loss supplements with no proven benefit. And you may have experienced the same financial frustration Carolyn felt after paying Weight Watchers dues for months only to regain all her lost weight. But does eating less (and eating well) and being more physically active actually cost more that the opposite tactic?

Take a close look at what you spend on food. If you're like the average

American, nearly half of your food budget goes toward away-from-home food. How many times per week do you eat at a sit-down restaurant? Consider spending the amount of just one restaurant receipt on fruits and vegetables instead. Contrary to popular belief, healthful foods don't necessarily cost more. Nutritious snacks are actually less expensive than unhealthful snacks, according to a 2006 article in *Today's Dietitian*. The authors compared the costs of nourishing and less nourishing choices in four categories: sweet snacks, salty snacks, high-fat and low-fat dips, and beverages. In all categories, the nourishing snacks were less expensive than the less nourishing versions. For example, the average price of eight varieties of fruit was 40 cents per serving, whereas the average price of foods such as brownies, pies, cookies, and sweet rolls was 53 cents per serving. Healthful salty snacks, like plain popcorn, peanuts, and pretzels, cost about 18 cents per serving. Beef jerky, fried pork rinds, cheese popcorn, and similar snacks cost nearly twice as much per serving.

Think about it: when you buy highly processed, packaged foods, you're paying a lot for the marketing and advertising and less for the food itself. A banana and a handful of raw almonds costs less than a nutrition bar and are just as convenient. Likewise, compare the price of bulk oatmeal (about 80 cents a pound) with a package of sweetened instant oatmeal, which is roughly five times as costly per serving.

What about exercise? Joining a gym and hiring a trainer can be pricey—even more so when you join and don't actually go. So think hard about whether you can make the commitment before signing a contract. For Carolyn, the investment was clearly worthwhile. But all you really need is a pair of comfortable shoes to get moving.

Now, consider the costs of staying at an unhealthy weight. To my mind, the physical and emotional toll of being overweight should be your primary concern. Be aware that overweight people who cannot stem their creeping weight gain may become obese. It may surprise you to know that obesity is a greater trigger for health problems and increased health spending than smoking or drinking. People who are obese have 30% to 50% more chronic medical problems than those who smoke or drink heavily.

CONCLUSION

I hope this book has inspired you to reset your set point, and more important, that it has given you the tools and knowledge to maintain your new, healthier weight. Once you become adept at tracking the different components of R-K-O, you can eventually shift over to writing down a single overall score that reflects the average of all your daily scores. After a while, you won't need to record a score because your newfound set point synergy will have become second nature. Whether you move from a silhouette 7 to a 6 and stay there indefinitely or drop from a silhouette 6 to a 3 over the course of several years, you will have succeeded.

Carolyn epitomizes the many patients who've participated in the dozens of clinical trials with which I've been involved in the past three decades. The findings from these studies—described in some four hundred scientific publications—combined with knowledge from the many experts I've quoted throughout the book, form the foundation of my advice, which is summarized in these five simple steps:

1. Eat less to weigh less.

2. Eat well to stay healthy.

3. Exercise to feel good.

4. Get sufficient sleep.

5. Control stress and enjoy life.

One key skill that makes all those steps possible is time management. Garner support from health care professionals, friends, family, and trainers. Gather your tools. Get inspired by programs in schools, workplaces, and your community. But in the end, it's all up to you. If a full-time working mother and single parent like Carolyn can do it, you can, too. Good luck.

Appendix

Chapter 4

Medical Interventions for Weight Loss

People who struggle with excess weight are often very interested in medical interventions—namely, drugs and surgery—to help them lose weight. Another option that appeals to some are medically supervised weight-loss programs, which typically combine behavioral-based treatment with weight-loss medications or surgery. Consult your primary care provider for a recommendation for a local program. Two examples are Health Management Resources (www.hmrprogram.com) and Optifast (www.optifast.com/optifast_home.do).

Medications

The Food and Drug Administration (FDA) has approved two prescription medications for long-term treatment of obesity: sibutramine and orlistat.

Sibutramine (Meridia) works by altering levels of chemicals in your brain that help control how full you feel. It doesn't suppress your appetite, but it may help you feel more satisfied with less food. In more than one hundred studies involving more than twelve thousand people, the average weight loss was 10 to 14 pounds over a year. Side effects include dry mouth, constipation, and insomnia. In some people, the drug causes blood pressure and heart rate to rise, so people who take this medication need to be monitored closely.

Orlistat (Xenical) targets the digestive system instead of the brain. It blocks about one-third of the fat in the food you eat from being absorbed by the body. The resulting side effects include loose stools, more frequent stools, and gas with oily discharge, particularly after high-fat meals. These unpleasant effects can help remind you to eat less fat, according to marketing materials for the product. An over-the-counter version of orlistat called Alli became available in June 2007. According to the Alli Web site (www.myalli.com), people who use this medication can lose 50% more weight than dieting alone (which means you could lose 15 pounds instead of 10).

Another novel class of weight-loss medications known as cannabinoid receptor blockers reduce appetite by blocking receptors in the brain that cause the munchies in marijuana users. One of these drugs, rimonabant also curbs nicotine cravings and has been proven to help people lose weight and quit smoking. Several studies show the drug can help improve cholesterol and other risk factors for heart disease. Although rimonabant, was approved in the United Kingdom in 2006, U.S. approval is pending and several pharmaceutical companies are working on similar drugs.

Doctors sometimes prescribe short-term weight loss medications, which are intended to be used for no longer than three months. These medications increase levels of norepinephrine (also known as noradrenaline), a brain chemical that helps regulate appetite and resting energy expenditure. Phentermine (Adipex-P, Ionamin, and others) is the safest. On average, people taking phentermine lose 2 to 13 pounds over a six-month period. After that, weight loss tends to level off, as it does with other diet drugs. Side effects include a rapid heartbeat and high blood pressure, nervousness, restlessness, and diarrhea.

Other Medications That Cause Weight Loss

Certain medications not specifically approved for weight loss may cause people to shed pounds. They include drugs used to treat diabetes, depression, and seizures. People who are overweight or obese who also have those medical conditions might consider asking their physicians about these medications, particularly if they are taking a related drug that might be contributing to their weight gain. (See the table of medications that may cause weight gain and some possible alternative medications.)

Surgery

Weight-loss surgery is considered only for people who have a BMI of 40 or more (severe obesity) who have had no success or only temporary success with other weight-loss approaches. People with mild to moderate obesity (a BMI between 30 and 39) may also be candidates for surgery if they have an obesity-related health problem, such as type 2 diabetes, heart disease, or sleep apnea. Currently, about 1% of people who are eligible for surgery choose to undergo one of the procedures.

The most common procedure, gastric bypass, used to require a large abdominal incision but is now done laparoscopically, which means the surgeon uses camera-guided instruments passed through tiny incisions. The surgeon converts the upper part of the stomach to a small pouch about the size of an egg and cuts the small intestine, connecting one end to the stomach pouch. The other end is reattached lower down, creating a **Y** shape.

A less common procedure (also done laparoscopically) is gastric banding. The surgeon places a 2-inch-wide silicone band around the top of the stomach to restrict the organ to a small upper section, with an opening at the bottom to the rest of the stomach and digestive tract. The size of the band can be adjusted by injecting or withdrawing saline (salt water) through a port implanted just under the skin.

With gastric bypass, patients usually lose up to half of their excess body weight in the first year after surgery. According to the Agency for Healthcare Quality and Research, gastric bypass accounts for the vast majority (94%) of weight-loss surgeries done in the United States. As a result, there is less information on the long-term effectiveness of the gastric band procedure. In general, people who get the band lose less weight and lose weight more slowly than those who undergo gastric bypass. But gastric banding surgery requires less time in the operating room, a shorter hospital stay, and fewer complications afterward. Gastric bypass, however, is now far less risky than in the past. In 1998, the risk of dying from the procedure was nearly 1 in 100. By 2004, the risk had dropped to 1 in 500.

As chair of the expert panel on weight-loss surgery at the Betsy Lehman Center for Patient Safety & Medical Error Reduction, I've been instrumental in shaping the panel's goals, which include identifying the best practices and clinical guidelines for the appropriate use of bariatric surgery and recommending specific steps to improve safety for people undergoing these procedures. The panel's recommendations have influenced surgery guidelines and standards in Massachusetts and other states.

The American Society for Bariatric Surgery and Surgical Review Corporation Centers of Excellence program represents a tandem effort to keep bariatric surgeries safe and effective by accrediting qualified hospitals and surgeons. This program increases patient safety by establishing best-practice guidelines and collecting data from qualified programs across the country. Currently, more than two hundred centers qualify as Centers of Excellence, with others being added regularly. To find those closest to you, go to the Surgical Review Corporation Web site (www.surgicalreview.org) and click on "Locate a Center of Excellence." From there, you can search by state, city, hospital, practice, or the surgeon's last name.

MEDICATIONS THAT MAY CAUSE WEIGHT GAIN
AND POSSIBLE ALTERNATIVES

Drug Class/Type	Generic Name	Trade Name	Alternative Drugs*	
Diabetes Treatments				
Insulin	insulin lispro	Humalog	metformin	Glucophage
			pramlintide	Symlin
Thiazolidenediones	rosiglitazone	Avandia	acarbose	Precose
	pioglitazone	Actos	miglitol	Glyset
DPP-4 inhibitors			sitagliptin	Januvia
			vildagliptin	Galvus
GLP-1 analogs			exenatide	Byetta
Sulfonylureas	glipizide	Glucotrol		
		Glucotrol XL		
	glyburide	Glynase		
	glimepiride	Amaryl		
Steroid Hormones				
Corticosteroids			NSAIDS	
Miscellaneous Agents				
Beta-adrenergic blockers	propranolol	Inderal	**ACE Inhibitors:**	
		Inderal LA	ramipril	Altace
	metoprolol	Lopressor	benazepril	Lotensin
		Toprol XL	enalapril	Vasotec
	atenolol	Tenormin	lisinopril	Prinivil
				Zestril
			Angiotensin II Receptor Blockers:	
			losartan	Cozaar
			candesartan	Atacand
			Calcium Channel Blockers:	
			amlodipine	Norvasc

*These medications have no effect on weight or may cause weight loss.

PSYCHIATRIC/NEUROLOGIC TREATMENTS

Antidepressants

Tricyclic antidepressants	amitriptyline	Elavil Vanatrip	bupropion	Wellbutrin Wellbutrin SR
	doxepin	Sinequan		Zyban
	imipramine	Tofranil	nefazodone	Serzone
	nortriptyline	Aventyl Pamelor		
	trimipramine	Surmontil		
	mirtazapine	Remeron		
Selective serotonin reuptake inhibitors (SSRIs)	paroxetine	Paxil	fluoxetine	Prozac
	fluvoxamine	Luvox	sertraline	Zoloft
	citalopram	Celexa		
	escitalopram	Lexapro		

Antipsychotics

	haloperidol	Haldol	ziprasidone	Geodon
	loxapine	Loxitane	aripiprazole	Abilify
	clozapine	Clozaril		
	olanzapine	Zyprexa		
	risperidone	Risperdal		
	quetiapine	Seroquel		

Anticonvulsants

	valproic acid (sodium valproate)	Depakote Depacon Depakene Depakote ER	topiramate zonisamide lamotrigine	Topamax Zonegran Lamictal
	carbamazepine	Carbatrol Epitol Tegretol Tegretol-XR		
	gabapentin	Neurontin		

BODY MASS INDEX FOR BMI 41–54

	41	42	43	44	45	46	47	48	49	50	51	52	53	54
Height							Weight in Pounds							
4'10"	196	201	205	210	215	220	224	229	234	239	244	248	253	258
4'11"	203	208	212	217	222	227	232	237	242	247	252	257	262	267
5'0"	209	215	220	225	230	235	240	245	250	255	261	266	271	276
5'1"	217	222	227	232	238	243	248	254	259	264	269	275	280	285
5'2"	224	229	235	240	246	251	256	262	267	273	278	284	289	295
5'3"	231	237	242	248	254	259	265	270	278	282	287	293	299	304
5'4"	238	244	250	256	262	267	273	279	285	291	296	302	308	314
5'5"	246	252	258	264	270	276	282	288	294	300	306	312	318	324
5'6"	253	260	266	272	278	284	291	297	303	309	315	322	328	334
5'7"	261	268	274	280	287	293	299	306	312	319	325	331	338	344
5'8"	269	276	282	289	295	302	308	315	322	328	335	341	348	354
5'9"	277	284	291	297	304	311	318	324	331	338	345	351	358	365
5'10"	285	292	299	306	313	320	327	334	341	348	355	362	369	376
5'11"	293	301	308	315	322	329	338	343	351	358	365	372	379	386
6'0"	302	309	316	324	331	338	346	353	361	368	375	383	390	397
6'1"	310	318	325	333	340	348	355	363	371	378	386	393	401	408
6'2"	319	326	334	342	350	358	365	373	381	389	396	404	412	420
6'3"	327	335	343	351	359	367	375	383	391	399	407	415	423	431
6'4"	336	344	353	361	369	377	385	394	402	410	418	426	435	443

Chapter 6

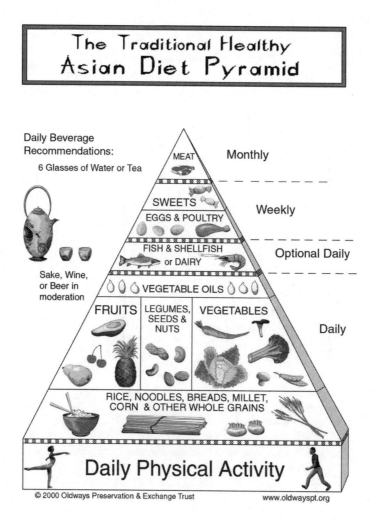

The Traditional Healthy Asian Diet Pyramid

Daily Beverage Recommendations:
6 Glasses of Water or Tea

Sake, Wine, or Beer in moderation

MEAT — Monthly

SWEETS
EGGS & POULTRY — Weekly

FISH & SHELLFISH or DAIRY — Optional Daily

VEGETABLE OILS

FRUITS | LEGUMES, SEEDS & NUTS | VEGETABLES — Daily

RICE, NOODLES, BREADS, MILLET, CORN & OTHER WHOLE GRAINS

Daily Physical Activity

© 2000 Oldways Preservation & Exchange Trust   www.oldwayspt.org

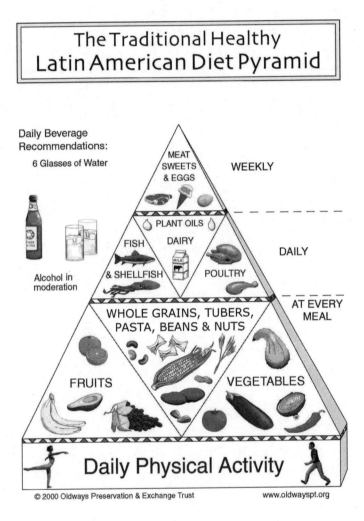

The Traditional Healthy
Latin American Diet Pyramid

Daily Beverage Recommendations:

6 Glasses of Water

Alcohol in moderation

MEAT SWEETS & EGGS   WEEKLY

PLANT OILS

FISH   DAIRY

& SHELLFISH   POULTRY   DAILY

WHOLE GRAINS, TUBERS, PASTA, BEANS & NUTS   AT EVERY MEAL

FRUITS   VEGETABLES

Daily Physical Activity

© 2000 Oldways Preservation & Exchange Trust   www.oldwayspt.org

The Traditional Healthy
Vegetarian Diet Pyramid

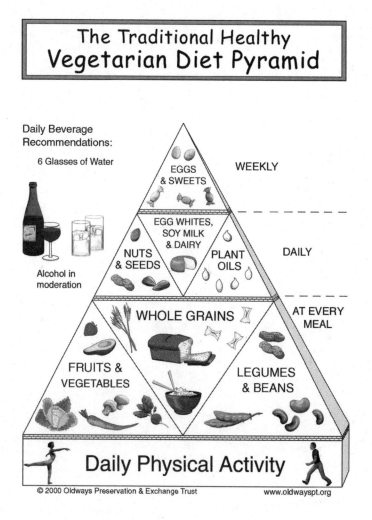

Daily Beverage Recommendations:

6 Glasses of Water

Alcohol in moderation

EGGS & SWEETS — WEEKLY

EGG WHITES, SOY MILK & DAIRY

NUTS & SEEDS

PLANT OILS — DAILY

WHOLE GRAINS — AT EVERY MEAL

FRUITS & VEGETABLES

LEGUMES & BEANS

Daily Physical Activity

© 2000 Oldways Preservation & Exchange Trust   www.oldwayspt.org

TUFTS

Food Guide Pyramid for Older Adults

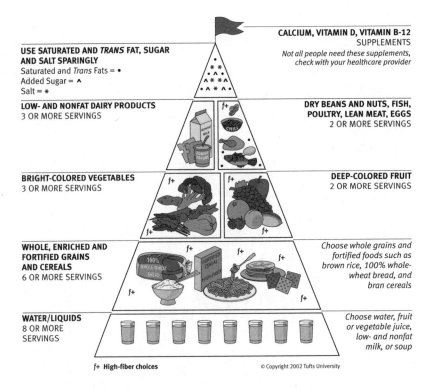

CALCIUM, VITAMIN D, VITAMIN B-12
SUPPLEMENTS
*Not all people need these supplements,
check with your healthcare provider*

**USE SATURATED AND *TRANS* FAT, SUGAR
AND SALT SPARINGLY**
Saturated and *Trans* Fats = •
Added Sugar = ^
Salt = *

LOW- AND NONFAT DAIRY PRODUCTS
3 OR MORE SERVINGS

**DRY BEANS AND NUTS, FISH,
POULTRY, LEAN MEAT, EGGS**
2 OR MORE SERVINGS

BRIGHT-COLORED VEGETABLES
3 OR MORE SERVINGS

DEEP-COLORED FRUIT
2 OR MORE SERVINGS

**WHOLE, ENRICHED AND
FORTIFIED GRAINS
AND CEREALS**
6 OR MORE SERVINGS

*Choose whole grains and
fortified foods such as
brown rice, 100% whole-
wheat bread, and
bran cereals*

WATER/LIQUIDS
8 OR MORE
SERVINGS

*Choose water, fruit
or vegetable juice,
low- and nonfat
milk, or soup*

f+ **High-fiber choices**   © Copyright 2002 Tufts University

For additional copies visit us on the web at **http://nutrition.tufts.edu**

HEALTHFUL PANTRY STAPLES

Foods to Look For	Tips
Fruit	
Fresh fruit Dried fruit	Buy a few extra apples or bananas to leave on your desk at work, as I do. They will keep for a few days and will help curb your cravings for an afternoon sweet. A great addition to cereal and salads, dried fruit can also help you meet your daily requirements of fruit.
Vegetables	
Fresh vegetables (spinach, broccoli) Frozen vegetables (corn, peas, carrots) Squash (butternut, acorn, pumpkin, zucchini, summer) Potatoes, sweet potatoes Onions, garlic	Check the frozen aisle for sales; stock up on marked-down vegetables to have on hand. Trying new and unusual vegetables is a great way to add some variety to your diet. Bok choy is great in stir-fries, while dark leafy greens like kale and Swiss chard are easily added to broth-based soups.
Grains, Beans, and Nuts	
Brown rice Oatmeal Whole-wheat pasta Ready-made whole-wheat pizza crust (you can find dough in the refrigerated section or already baked in the bread aisle) Whole-wheat pita bread Barley, couscous, quinoa Beans (canned or dry) Almonds	Grains like barley, couscous, and quinoa are great to have on hand because they keep indefinitely. You can always use them to add a little fiber and protein to soups, stews, and casseroles. Try mixing them with cut-up vegetables and a little olive oil, then chilling, for another take on pasta salad. Not only are beans a great source of protein, but they are incredibly versatile as well. Lentils are a great choice, because they cook up quickly and don't need to be soaked overnight. For the best value, try looking for nuts in the bulk aisle or at a superstore like Costco or Sam's Club. Try roasting unsalted nuts in the toaster oven for a quick snack.

(continued)

Meat, Poultry, and Fish	
Lean meat Skinless, boneless chicken breasts Fresh fish	Look for beef with the word *loin* or *round* in the name (top round, tenderloin, etc.). If you're buying ground beef, ground round is the leanest.
Dairy	
Milk Cheese Eggs Yogurt Cottage cheese	Remember to choose low- or nonfat dairy. Cottage cheese is a great source of protein. Eat it on its own, topped with fruit, or in a salad.
Other Staples	
Low-sodium chicken or vegetable stock Tomato sauce Spices	Spices are the key to a tasty, savory meal. Keep a variety of your favorites on hand to add flavor to sautés, casseroles, soups, or even simple steamed vegetables.

Meal and Menu Planning

The following are menu ideas and recipes, as well as a few dessert recipes. Remember that you want to try to eat at least 450 calories at breakfast and lunch, so supplement the lower-calorie recipes (e.g., Fruit Smoothie and Berry Parfait) with two slices of whole-grain toast with a teaspoon of margarine (about 200 calories). Or try the menu ideas, which contain approximately 450 calories.

BREAKFAST
● ● ● ● ● ● ●

#1
1 cup Multi-Bran Chex Cereal
1 cup nonfat milk
½ cup strawberry halves
1 whole-grain English muffin
1 tsp. margarine

#2
1 poached or soft-boiled egg
6 oz. nonfat vanilla yogurt mixed with
    ¼ cup fresh/frozen blueberries
2 slices whole-wheat toast
1 tsp. margarine

#3
1 cup plain oatmeal
1 cup fresh/frozen berries
1 tbsp. walnuts (7 walnut halves)
2 tsp. brown sugar
1 cup nonfat milk

RECIPES
● ● ● ● ●

FRUIT SMOOTHIE
Serves 4

2 bananas
16 medium strawberries
2 medium kiwis
1 cup nonfat plain yogurt
1½ cups orange juice
2 tsp. wheat germ
1 cup ice

Place all ingredients in a blender and blend until smooth.

Calories per serving: 171

TOASTED PEANUT BUTTER
AND BANANA SANDWICH
Serves 4

8 slices whole-wheat bread
½ cup peanut butter
2 medium bananas, sliced
4 tsp. honey

Toast the bread. For each of the four sandwiches, spread 2 tablespoons of peanut butter on one slice of bread. Layer banana slices evenly over the peanut butter and drizzle each sandwich with 1 teaspoon of honey. Top each sandwich with another slice of bread.

Calories per serving: 460

APRICOT WALNUT OATMEAL

Serves 4

4 cups nonfat milk
2 cups old-fashioned rolled oats
2 tbsp. apricot jam
2 tbsp. chopped walnuts
¼ cup chopped dried apricots (optional)

Bring the milk to a slow boil in a saucepan. Stir in the oats and cook for about 5 minutes, stirring occasionally. Once the oatmeal is cooked, swirl in the apricot jam. Sprinkle with walnuts and dried apricots.

Calories per serving: 319 (241 without apricots)

STRAWBERRY BANANA OAT SMOOTHIE

Serves 4

2 medium bananas
28 medium strawberries
2 tbsp. honey
2 cups nonfat milk
1 tsp. vanilla extract
2 tbsp. oat bran

Place all ingredients in a blender and blend until smooth.

Calories per serving: 164

SCRAMBLED SALSA BREAKFAST BURRITO

Serves 4

8 large eggs
2 tbsp. nonfat milk
½ tsp. salt

½ tsp. pepper
1 tbsp. olive oil
1 cup shredded low-fat cheddar cheese
four 10-inch whole-wheat tortillas
1 cup salsa
hot sauce (optional)

Beat the eggs, milk, salt, and pepper in a bowl and set aside. Heat the olive oil in a nonstick pan over medium-high heat. Add the egg mixture to the olive oil and scramble. Add the cheese before the eggs are finished cooking, about 3 minutes. Remove the eggs from the heat after they are fully cooked.

Place the tortillas in damp paper towels and microwave for 30 seconds. Spread one-quarter of the salsa and hot sauce, if desired, in a line down the center of each tortilla. Divide the scrambled eggs evenly among the tortillas and roll each one into a burrito.

Calories per serving: 449

BERRY PARFAIT
Serves 4

3 cups nonfat vanilla or plain yogurt (¾ cup per serving)
1 cup low-fat granola (¼ cup per serving)
1 cup berries of choice
4 tsp. honey
other fruit such as sliced bananas or peaches (optional)

For each serving, put about half of the yogurt in the bottom of a bowl, sprinkle some granola and berries, then add the rest of the yogurt. Top with the remaining granola and fruit, and drizzle each serving with 1 teaspoon of honey.

Calories per serving: 249

LUNCH
• • • • •

#1
Mexican-Style Wrap
1 orange

#2
Chef Salad
2 Wasa multigrain crisp bread crackers
1 medium apple

#3
1 cup garden vegetable soup (Healthy Choice)
Roast beef sandwich (whole-wheat bun, 2 oz. lean roast beef deli meat,
    1 slice low-fat Swiss cheese, mustard, romaine lettuce)
1 plum
8 oz. nonfat milk

RECURPES

● ● ● ● ●

CHEF SALAD
Serves 4

8 cups romaine lettuce, torn into small pieces
8 oz. 95% lean turkey meat
8 oz. 97% lean ham
2 oz. low-fat cheese
1 tomato, sliced
6 tbsp. low-fat balsamic vinaigrette dressing

Toss the lettuce with the turkey, ham, cheese, and tomato. Drizzle the dressing over the top and serve.

Calories per serving: 203

PASTA FASZULI
Serves 4

½ pound whole-wheat elbow pasta
14 oz. canned crushed tomatoes
½ tsp. garlic powder
½ tsp. pepper
½ tsp. oregano
8 oz. canned red kidney beans
1 tbsp. Parmesan cheese

Cook the pasta according to the package directions. Meanwhile, simmer the crushed tomatoes, garlic powder, pepper, and oregano in a saucepan for 15 minutes. Add the kidney beans with their liquid, and continue to simmer until heated through. After the pasta is cooked, drain it and toss it with the sauce. Sprinkle with the Parmesan and serve.

Calories per serving: 314

VEGETABLE FRITTATA
Serves 4

8 eggs
1 tsp. salt
1 tsp. pepper
1 cup grated part-skim mozzarella cheese
1 tbsp. olive oil
½ onion, sliced
1 red pepper, sliced
1 yellow pepper, sliced
1½ cups mushrooms, sliced
1 summer squash, sliced

Preheat the oven to 350°F. Beat the eggs, adding the salt and pepper. Stir in the mozzarella cheese and set aside. Heat the olive oil in a nonstick ovenproof skillet, and sauté the onions over medium heat until they start to look translucent, about 2 minutes. Add the peppers and mushrooms, and cook until they become tender, about 2 minutes. Add the squash and cook for another 2 minutes. Pour the egg mixture over the vegetables, and cook for about 10 minutes, until the eggs have set around the edges. Transfer the skillet to the oven and cook for another 10 to 15 minutes, until the eggs are completely set and a fork comes out clean. Slice into wedges and serve immediately.

Calories per serving: 300

MEXICAN-STYLE WRAP
Serves 4

1 tbsp. olive oil
½ onion, sliced

1 green pepper, sliced
1 red pepper, sliced
1 orange pepper, sliced
16 oz. canned low-fat refried beans
½ avocado, sliced
½ tomato, diced
½ cup salsa
four 10-inch whole-wheat flour tortillas
½ jalapeño pepper, seeded and chopped (optional)

Heat the olive oil in a nonstick skillet over medium-high heat. Add the onions and peppers (including jalapeño, if used) and sauté until tender, then set aside in a bowl. Add the refried beans to the warm skillet and stir over medium heat until heated through, then set aside. Make a simple guacamole sauce by mashing the avocado and tomato together in a bowl.

Spread one-quarter of the beans, one-quarter of the peppers and onions, one-quarter of the guacamole, and 2 tablespoons of the salsa on each tortilla. Roll each tortilla into a wrap.

Calories per serving: 444

TOASTED HARD-BOILED EGG SANDWICH

Serves 4

8 large hard-boiled eggs, chopped
2 tomatoes, diced
salt
pepper
dried parsley
8 slices whole-wheat bread
4 slices low-fat Swiss cheese

Mix the eggs and tomatoes in a bowl. Add the salt, pepper, and parsley to taste. Toast the bread. For each sandwich, spread one-quarter of the egg and tomato filling onto one slice of the bread, add one slice of cheese, and top with another slice of bread.

Calories per serving: 396

CRANBERRY CHICKEN SALAD SANDWICH
Serves 4

four 3-oz. skinless, boneless chicken breasts, baked and shredded
¼ cup light mayonnaise
1 cup dried cranberries or red grapes, halved
¼ cup sliced almonds
salt
pepper
8 slices whole-wheat bread
4 leaves green-leaf lettuce

Mix the chicken, mayonnaise, cranberries (or grapes), and almonds together in a bowl. Add salt and pepper to taste. For each sandwich, spread one-quarter of the chicken filling onto one slice of bread, add a lettuce leaf, and top with another slice of bread.

Calories per serving: 423

DINNER

For dinner, follow my plate management suggestion: one-half vegetables, one-quarter starchy vegetable or grain, and one-quarter protein. To keep it simple, you can pick your favorite protein (fish, tofu, chicken, lean beef or pork), then add a serving of grains and two servings of vegetables.

#1
Asian Salmon Packets
Whole-Wheat Couscous
Lemon Parmesan Asparagus
Blueberry and Lemon Crumble

#2
Chicken Cacciatore
Brown Rice
Sautéed Broccoli
Warm Apples with Ice Cream

#3
Spice-Rubbed Flank Steak
Baked Potato Wedges
Garlic Spinach
Fresh fruit

#4
Texas Turkey Chili
Whole-wheat rolls or corn bread
Green salad (mixed greens with low-fat dressing)
Fresh fruit sorbet

#5
Barbeque Pizza
Chocolate-covered Strawberries

RECITES

● ● ● ● ●

ASIAN SALMON PACKETS
Serves 4

four 3- to 4-oz. salmon fillets
¼ cup reduced-sodium soy sauce
2 tbsp. lemon juice
2 tsp. minced fresh ginger
2 tsp. sesame oil
1 tbsp. toasted sesame seeds
slivered green onions, mushrooms, and sliced peppers (optional)

Preheat the oven to 400°F. Cut four 12-by-12-inch squares of parchment paper or aluminum foil. Place one salmon fillet in the middle of each square. Mix the soy sauce, lemon juice, ginger, sesame oil, and sesame seeds in a bowl. Divide this mixture evenly and pour over the fillets. If desired, add the onions, mushrooms, and peppers. Seal each packet (if you are using foil, simply bring the edges together and fold; if you are using parchment paper, bring the edges together, fold, and seal with a stapler). Place the packets on a baking sheet and bake for 10 minutes, or until fish is done.

Calories per serving: 219

CHICKEN CACCIATORE
Serves 8

2 lb. boneless chicken breasts, cubed
1 cup chopped onion
1 cup chopped zucchini
1 cup chopped red pepper
1 cup chopped green pepper
½ cup chopped mushrooms
28 oz. canned crushed tomatoes
½ tsp. pepper
½ tsp. garlic powder
1 tbsp. Italian seasoning

Preheat the oven to 350°F. Place all the ingredients in an oven bag and mix them well. Poke a few holes in the bag and place it in a 9-by-13-inch baking pan. Bake the chicken for 45 minutes.

Calories per serving: 175

BARBECUE PIZZA
Serves 4

10 oz. whole-wheat pizza crust (available as dough in the refrigerated section of your supermarket or already baked in the bakery aisle)
⅓ cup barbecue sauce
½ cup corn kernels (fresh or frozen)
1 cup canned black beans, rinsed and drained
½ green pepper, diced
1 tomato, diced
¼ red onion, thinly sliced
1 cup shredded Monterey Jack cheese
2 tbsp. chopped fresh cilantro
grilled chicken breast, cubed (optional)

Preheat the oven to 450°F. Stretch out the pizza dough into a 12-inch-diameter circle and place on a lightly greased pizza pan. Spread the barbecue sauce evenly over the dough. Sprinkle the rest of the toppings on the pizza. Bake for 10 minutes, or until the crust is golden brown and the cheese is melted.

Note: The baking directions for your pizza dough may be slightly different; follow those for best results. (Adapted from "Eating Well," http://www.eatingwell.com/recipes/corn_black_bean_pizza.html.)

Calories per serving: 478 without chicken breast; 540 with 2 oz. chicken breast

SPICE-RUBBED FLANK STEAK
Serves 4

2 tsp. chili powder
1 tsp. cumin
1 tsp. pepper
1 tsp. brown sugar
½ tsp. oregano
½ tsp. cayenne pepper
1 lb. flank steak

Combine the spices and rub all over both sides of the flank steak. Wrap the meat in plastic and refrigerate 1 to 2 hours or overnight.

Grill the steak on a lightly oiled rack, 5 to 8 minutes on each side for medium rare. Or roll the flank steak and secure it with two skewers. Preheat the oven to 350°F. Place the steak in a baking pan and cook for approximately 45 to 55 minutes. (Meat is done when it is slightly pink in the center; use a knife to check.) Remove skewers and slice across the grain of the meat.

Calories per serving: 241

TEXAS TURKEY CHILI
Serves 8–10 (you can take leftovers for lunch or freeze)

1 tbsp. olive or canola oil
1 small white onion, diced
1 tsp. minced garlic
1 tsp. red chili pepper flakes
1 tbsp. chili powder
1 lb. ground turkey meat, lean
32 oz. canned kidney beans, rinsed and drained
28 oz. canned diced tomatoes
3 oz. tomato paste

1 green pepper, diced
1 cup frozen vegetables (corn, carrots)
Tabasco sauce

In a large soup pot, sauté the oil, onions, garlic, pepper flakes, and chili powder over medium heat. Add the turkey and sauté until cooked through. Turn the heat to low and add the beans, tomatoes, tomato paste, peppers, and vegetables. Simmer, uncovered, on low heat for 30 to 40 minutes. Season with Tabasco, chili flakes, and chili powder to obtain the desired flavor.

Calories per serving: 281

VEGETABLES
● ● ● ● ● ● ● ●

SAUTÉED BROCCOLI
Serves 4

1 tbsp. vegetable oil
1 tsp. sesame oil
1 clove garlic, chopped
4 cups broccoli florets
salt

Heat the vegetable and sesame oils in a skillet over medium heat. Add the garlic and stir until golden. Add the broccoli florets and sauté until the broccoli is crisp-tender and bright green, stirring often. Add salt to taste.

Calories per serving: 62

GARLIC SPINACH
Serves 4

1 tsp. olive oil
1 garlic clove, chopped
12 oz. fresh baby spinach
salt
pepper

Heat the oil and garlic in a skillet over medium-high heat. Add the spinach. Stir often, cooking for 1 to 2 minutes or until just wilted. Add salt and pepper to taste.

Note: For more variety, try adding one or more of the following: 1 to 2 tbsp. chopped, toasted walnuts or pine nuts; 1 to 2 tbsp. crumbled feta or Gorgonzola cheese; 1 to 2 tbsp. dried cranberries or raisins; a few dashes of olive oil or balsamic vinaigrette dressing.

Calories per serving: 30

GLAZED CARROTS
Serves 4

2 cups baby carrots
2 tbsp. honey
2 tbsp. butter or margarine
¼ tsp. nutmeg
2 tsp. dried basil

Boil water in a saucepan. Add the carrots and cook, covered, for 7 to 10 minutes or until barely tender. Drain the carrots and set aside. Add the honey, butter, nutmeg, and basil to the warm saucepan and stir over medium heat until the ingredients are combined and the butter is melted. Return the carrots to the saucepan and cook for another 2 minutes.
Calories per serving: 108

LEMON PARMESAN ASPARAGUS
Serves 4

1 bunch asparagus (about 1 lb.)
1 tbsp. olive oil
1 tbsp. lemon juice
½ tsp. salt
½ tsp. ground pepper
2 tbsp. Parmesan cheese

Preheat the oven to 400°F. Spread the asparagus on a baking sheet. Drizzle the olive oil, lemon juice, salt, and pepper over the asparagus stalks. Roast in the oven for 15 minutes or until tender. Sprinkle with the cheese.

Calories per serving: 70

GREEN BEANS WITH BALSAMIC VINAIGRETTE
Serves 4

1½ tsp. salt, divided
1 lb. fresh green beans, trimmed
1 shallot, chopped
2 tbsp. balsamic vinegar
1 tbsp. olive oil
½ tsp. pepper

Bring a large pot of water and a teaspoon of salt to a boil. Add the green beans and cook for 5 to 7 minutes or until crisp-tender. After draining, plunge the green beans into a bowl of ice water to prevent further cooking. In a bowl, whisk the chopped shallots, balsamic vinegar, olive oil, remaining salt, and pepper together. Drain the green beans and toss them with the dressing in a large bowl.

Calories per serving: 75

GRAINS AND STARCHY VEGETABLES

BAKED POTATO WEDGES
Serves 4

2 large russet (about 1¼ lb.) potatoes
2 tbsp. olive oil
salt
pepper

Preheat the oven to 400°F. Slice each potato into thin wedges. Spread, one layer thick, on foil that has been brushed with olive oil. Brush olive oil lightly over the tops of the wedges. Bake for 10 minutes, then flip the wedges over. Sprinkle salt and pepper over the wedges and bake for another 10 to 20 minutes, or until the potatoes are done.

Calories per serving: 202

BROWN RICE
Serves 4

1 cup uncooked brown rice

Boil 2 cups of water in a saucepan. Add the rice, cover, and simmer on low heat for 40 to 45 minutes.

Calories per serving: 172

WHOLE-WHEAT COUSCOUS

Serves 4

1 tsp. olive oil
salt
½ cup whole-wheat couscous

Bring two-thirds of a cup of water to a boil, adding the olive oil and a dash of salt. Stir in the couscous, cover the pan, and remove it from the heat. After 5 minutes, uncover the pan and fluff the couscous with a fork.

Calories per serving: 91

HERBED BULGUR WHEAT

Serves 4

1 cup bulgur wheat
salt
2½ cups water, or chicken or vegetable stock
1 tbsp. olive oil
salt
pepper
chopped fresh parsley, basil, or chives (optional)

Measure 1 cup of bulgur in a bowl with a pinch of salt and add 2½ cups of boiling water or chicken or vegetable stock. Cover the pot and let stand for 25 minutes (15 minutes if using fine bulgur). Toss with the olive oil and salt and pepper to taste. Add a little chopped parsley or other chopped herbs, such as basil or chives, if desired.

Note: Bulgur is steamed, cracked whole-wheat kernels. Like brown rice, you can buy it in bulk bins and in packages.

Calories per serving: 204

CORN WITH AVOCADO-LIME SALSA
Serves 4

2 cups cooked corn kernels (or frozen and defrosted corn)
½ avocado, diced
½ red onion, chopped
¼ cup chopped fresh cilantro
juice of one lime
½ cup halved grape or cherry tomatoes
½ tsp. cumin
salt
pepper

Mix all the ingredients together in a bowl, and add salt and pepper to taste. Chill before serving.

Calories per serving: 141

DESSERTS
● ● ● ● ● ● ●

BLUEBERRY AND LEMON CRUMBLE
Serves 8

4 cups blueberries, fresh or frozen
¼ cup brown sugar
1 tbsp. flour
1 tsp. lemon juice
2 tsp. freshly grated lemon zest

Crumble topping:
1 cup flour
⅔ cup brown sugar
1 tsp. cinnamon
salt
½ cup butter

Preheat the oven to 350°F. Place the berries in a greased 8-by-8-inch baking dish. Mix with the brown sugar, flour, lemon juice, and lemon zest. To make the topping, blend the flour, brown sugar, cinnamon, and salt in a bowl; then add the butter and mix with a fork. Sprinkle the topping evenly over the berries. Bake for 20 to 30 minutes, or until the berries are bubbling and the crumble topping is golden brown. Serve warm.

Calories per serving: 291

WARM APPLES WITH ICE CREAM
Serves 4

1 tbsp. butter
4 apples, cored and sliced
2 tbsp. brown sugar
1 tsp. cinnamon
1 tbsp. lemon juice
2 cups low-fat vanilla ice cream

Melt the butter in a pan over medium heat. Add the apples, brown sugar, cinnamon, and lemon juice. Sauté, stirring often, until the apples are tender. Serve over low-fat vanilla ice cream.

Calories per serving: 250

CHOCOLATE-COVERED STRAWBERRIES
Serves 6

6 oz. semisweet chocolate chips
1 lb. strawberries, stems intact

Line a baking sheet with parchment or waxed paper. Melt the chocolate chips over a double boiler or in the microwave, stirring often. When the chocolate is melted, remove from the heat. Dip each strawberry two-thirds of the way into the chocolate, then place on the baking sheet. After all the strawberries have been dipped, let them sit until the chocolate hardens. You can also chill them in the refrigerator.

Calories per serving: 156

Recommended Cookbooks
Fit Food: Eating Well for Life
Ellen Haas
Ellen Haas, former undersecretary of agriculture for Food, Nutrition, and Consumer Services, is a leading expert in the field of healthful eating, and

her cookbooks provide delicious and sensible recipes and tips. *Fit Food* captures the highlights of the nutrition information available on her Web site, www.foodfit.com, which I also highly recommend. *Fit Food* includes recipes by such nationally recognized chefs as Alice Waters, Jody Adams, and Todd English.

Diabetes Fit Food
Ellen Haas
Following the success of *Fit Food,* Ellen Haas released a version with recipes and tips tailored specifically to the needs of the diabetic.

The New American Plate Cookbook: Recipes for a Healthy Weight and a Healthy Life
American Institute for Cancer Research
Based on the AICR's approach to plate management (see Chapter 6), *The New American Plate Cookbook* includes two hundred delicious recipes that emphasize grains, vegetables, fruits, and beans. The book also includes all the necessary nutritional information, making it easy to regulate portion size.

Vegetarian Cooking for Everyone
Deborah Madison
Chock full of recipes and tips, this is a go-to book for me and many of my staff. Deborah Madison provides the reader with simple recipes for both well-known and obscure vegetables and meatless ingredients. This book can serve as a manual for how to select, prepare, and cook your ingredients. Not just for vegetarians, many of the book's recipes can be easily modified to include meat.

American Heart Association Quick & Easy Cookbook: More Than 200 Healthful Recipes You Can Make in Minutes
American Heart Association
This volume offers a variety of tasty, healthful recipes, most of which take only thirty minutes to prepare. All recipes include preparation and cooking time, as well as nutritional information.

Eating Well Serves Two: 150 Healthy in a Hurry Suppers
Jim Romanoff, The Test Kitchen of Eating Well *Magazine*
I like this book for its simple, healthy recipes and tips for the two-person household. *Eating Well Serves Two* includes a guide about strategies for shopping for, storing, and easily cooking smaller quantities without wasting food.

Chapter 7

GENERAL PHYSICAL ACTIVITIES DEFINED BY LEVEL OF INTENSITY (IN ACCORDANCE WITH CDC AND ACSM GUIDELINES)*

Moderate Activity* (3.5 to 7 kcal/min)	Vigorous Activity* (more than 7 kcal/min)
Walking at a moderate or brisk pace of 3 to 4.5 mph on a level surface inside or outside, such as walking to class, work, or the store; walking for pleasure; walking the dog; or walking as a break from work. Walking downstairs or down a hill Racewalking—less than 5 mph Using crutches Hiking Roller skating or in-line skating at a leisurely pace	Racewalking and aerobic walking—5 mph or faster Jogging or running Wheeling your wheelchair Walking and climbing briskly up a hill Backpacking Mountain climbing, rock climbing, or rappeling Roller skating or in-line skating at a brisk pace
Bicycling 5 to 9 mph, level terrain, or with few hills Stationary bicycling—using moderate effort	Bicycling more than 10 mph or bicycling on steep uphill terrain Stationary bicycling—with vigorous effort
Aerobic dancing—low impact Water aerobics	Aerobic dancing—high impact Step aerobics Water jogging Teaching an aerobic dance class
Calisthenics—light Yoga	Calisthenics—push-ups, pull-ups, vigorous effort

Moderate Activity* (3.5 to 7 kcal/min)	Vigorous Activity* (more than 7 kcal/min)
Gymnastics General home exercises, light or moderate effort, getting up and down from the floor Jumping on a trampoline Using a stair climber machine at a light-to-moderate pace Using a rowing machine—with moderate effort	Karate, judo, tae kwon do, jujitsu Jumping rope Performing jumping jacks Using a stair climber machine at a fast pace Using a rowing machine—with vigorous effort Using an arm cycling machine—with vigorous effort
Weight training and bodybuilding using free weights, Nautilus- or Universal-type weights	Circuit weight training
Boxing—punching bag	Boxing—in the ring, sparring Wrestling—competitive
Ballroom dancing Line dancing Square dancing Folk dancing Modern dancing, disco Ballet	Professional ballroom dancing—energetically Square dancing—energetically Folk dancing—energetically Clogging
Table tennis—competitive Tennis—doubles	Tennis—singles Wheelchair tennis
Golf, wheeling or carrying clubs	—
Softball—fast pitch or slow pitch Basketball—shooting baskets Coaching children's or adults' sports	Most competitive sports Football game Basketball game Wheelchair basketball Soccer Rugby Kickball Field or in-line hockey Lacrosse
Volleyball—competitive	Beach volleyball—on sand court
Playing Frisbee Juggling Curling Cricket—batting and bowling Badminton Archery (nonhunting) Fencing	Handball—general or team Racquetball Squash

(continued)

GENERAL PHYSICAL ACTIVITIES DEFINED BY LEVEL
OF INTENSITY (IN ACCORDANCE WITH CDC
AND ACSM GUIDELINES)* *(continued)*

Moderate Activity* (3.5 to 7 kcal/min)	Vigorous Activity* (more than 7 kcal/min)
Downhill skiing—with light effort Ice-skating at a leisurely pace (9 mph or less) Snowmobiling Ice sailing	Downhill skiing—racing or with vigorous effort Ice-skating—fast pace or speed skating Cross-country skiing Sledding Tobogganing Playing ice hockey
Swimming—recreational Treading water—slowly, moderate effort Diving—springboard or platform Aquatic aerobics Waterskiing Snorkeling Surfing, board or body	Swimming—steady paced laps Synchronized swimming Treading water—fast, vigorous effort Water jogging Water polo Water basketball Scuba diving
Canoeing or rowing a boat at less than 4 mph Rafting—whitewater Sailing—recreational or competitive Paddle boating Kayaking—on a lake, calm water Washing or waxing a powerboat or the hull of a sailboat	Canoeing or rowing—4 or more mph Kayaking in whitewater rapids
Fishing while walking along a riverbank or while wading in a stream—wearing waders	—
Hunting deer, large or small game Pheasant and grouse hunting Hunting with a bow and arrow or crossbow—walking	—
Horseback riding—general Saddling or grooming a horse	Horseback riding—trotting, galloping, jumping, or in competition Playing polo

Moderate Activity* (3.5 to 7 kcal/min)	Vigorous Activity* (more than 7 kcal/min)
Playing on school playground equipment, moving about, swinging, or climbing Playing hopscotch, 4-square, dodgeball, T-ball, or tetherball Skateboarding Roller-skating or in-line skating—leisurely pace	Running Skipping Jumping rope Performing jumping jacks Roller-skating or in-line skating—fast pace
Playing instruments while actively moving; playing in a marching band; playing guitar or drums in a rock band Twirling a baton in a marching band Singing while actively moving about—as on stage or in church	Playing a heavy musical instrument while actively running in a marching band
Gardening and yard work: raking the lawn, bagging grass or leaves, digging, hoeing, light shoveling (less than 10 lb. per minute), or weeding while standing or bending Planting trees, trimming shrubs and trees, hauling branches, stacking wood Pushing a power lawn mower or tiller	Gardening and yard work: heavy or rapid shoveling (more than 10 lb. per minute), digging ditches, or carrying heavy loads Felling trees, carrying large logs, swinging an ax, hand-splitting logs, or climbing and trimming trees Pushing a nonmotorized lawn mower
Shoveling light snow	Shoveling heavy snow
Moderate housework: scrubbing the floor or bathtub while on hands and knees, hanging laundry on a clothesline, sweeping an outdoor area, cleaning out the garage, washing windows, moving light furniture, packing or unpacking boxes, walking and putting household items away, carrying out heavy bags of trash or recyclables (e.g., glass, newspapers, and plastics), or carrying water or firewood General household tasks requiring considerable effort	Heavy housework: moving or pushing heavy furniture (75 lb. or more), carrying household items weighing 25 lb. or more up a flight of stairs, or shoveling coal into a stove Standing, walking, or walking down a flight of stairs while carrying objects weighing 50 lb. or more

(*continued*)

GENERAL PHYSICAL ACTIVITIES DEFINED BY LEVEL OF INTENSITY (IN ACCORDANCE WITH CDC AND ACSM GUIDELINES)* *(continued)*

Moderate Activity* (3.5 to 7 kcal/min)	Vigorous Activity* (more than 7 kcal/min)
Putting groceries away—walking and carrying especially large items less than 50 lb.	Carrying several heavy bags (25 lb. or more) of groceries at one time up a flight of stairs Grocery shopping while carrying young children and pushing a full grocery cart, or pushing two full grocery carts at once
Actively playing with children—walking, running, or climbing while playing with children Walking while carrying a child weighing less than 50 lb. Walking while pushing or pulling a child in a stroller or an adult in a wheelchair Carrying a child weighing less than 25 lb. up a flight of stairs Child care: handling uncooperative young children (e.g., chasing, dressing, lifting into car seat), or handling several young children at one time Bathing and dressing an adult	Vigorously playing with children—running longer distances or playing strenuous games with children Racewalking or jogging while pushing a stroller designed for sport use Carrying someone weighing 25 lb. or more up a flight of stairs Standing or walking while carrying someone weighing 50 lb. or more

Source: U.S. Department of Health and Human Services, Public Health Service, Centers for Disease Control and Prevention, National Center for Chronic Disease Prevention and Health Promotion, Division of Nutrition and Physical Activity. *Promoting Physical Activity: A Guide for Community Action.* Champaign, IL: Human Kinetics, 1999.

* For an average person, defined here as 70 kilograms or 154 pounds. The activity intensity levels portrayed in this chart are most applicable to men 30 to 50 years old and women 20 to 40 years old. For older individuals, the classification of activity intensity might be higher. For example, what is moderate intensity to a 40-year-old man might be vigorous for a man in his 70s. Intensity is a subjective classification.

ACTIVITY CONVERTED TO STEPS

Activity	Steps per Minute	
	Female	Male
Aerobic dancing (low impact)	142	127
Aerobics (high impact)	189	181

Activity	Steps per Minute	
	Female	Male
Aerobics step 6–8 inch step	236	218
Aerobics step 10–12 inch step	260	254
Backpacking on hill with under 10 lb. load	189	181
Backpacking on hill with under 10–20 lb. load	212	199
Ballet dancing	118	127
Baseball	142	127
Basketball (leisurely, nongame)	165	127
Basketball (game)	212	145
Basketball (playing in wheelchair)	165	163
Bicycling	212	199
Bicycling (BMX or mountain)	236	218
Bicycling—stationary—general	189	181
Bicycling—stationary—light	142	145
Bicycling—stationary—moderate	189	181
Bicycling—stationary—vigorous	283	254
Bowling	71	73
Canoeing	94	91
Chopping wood	165	145
Circuit training (general)	212	199
Dancing ballroom (slow)	71	73
Dancing ballroom (fast)	118	109
Dancing country, disco, line, square, or swing	118	109
Elliptical jogger (medium)	236	218
Football tackle	236	218
Football touch/flag	212	199

(*continued*)

ACTIVITY CONVERTED TO STEPS *(continued)*

	Steps per Minute	
Activity	Female	Male
Gardening (moderate)	118	109
Gardening (heavy)	142	145
Golfing (without cart)	118	109
Golfing (riding in cart)	94	91
Horseshoes	71	73
Ice skating (leisurely)	189	181
In-line skating	200	190
Jogging (general)	189	181
Jogging (in water)	212	199
Judo and karate	260	254
Jumping rope (slow)	212	199
Jumping rope (moderate)	260	254
Jumping rope (fast)	330	290
Kickboxing (moderate)	330	290
Kickboxing (vigorous)	401	363
Kickboxing (very vigorous)	472	435
Mowing lawn	142	127
Pilates	94	91
Racquetball (casual)	189	181
Racquetball (competitive)	260	254
Rowing	189	181
Running 8 mph (7.5 min./mile)	354	326
Running 10 mph (6 min./mile)	425	399
Scrubbing floors	94	91
Shoveling snow	165	145

Activity	Steps per Minute	
	Female	Male
Skiing downhill (moderate to steep)	165	145
Skiing cross-country	212	181
Snowshoeing	212	199
Soccer (casual)	189	181
Soccer (competitive)	260	145
Stair climber machine	236	218
Stair climbing—up stairs	212	199
Stair climbing—down stairs	71	73
Swimming backstroke	189	181
Swimming breaststroke	260	254
Swimming butterfly	283	272
Swimming freestyle	189	181
Swimming sidestroke	212	199
Tennis (singles)	212	199
Tennis (doubles)	165	145
Vacuuming	94	73
Volleyball	118	91
Walking	94	91
Washing the car	71	73
Waterskiing	165	145
Waxing the car	118	109
Weight lifting	71	73
Wrestling	165	145
Yoga	71	54

Source: Copyright © 2005, America On the Move Foundation. Used with permission from The America On the Move Foundation, Inc. For more information, please visit www.americaonthemove.org.

Chapter 8
PLANNING AHEAD USING A DAY PLANNER

Time	To Do	Hours	Why
5:00 A.M.			
6:00 A.M.			
7:00 A.M.			
8:00 A.M.			
9:00 A.M.			
10:00 A.M.			
11:00 A.M.			
Noon			
1:00 P.M.			
2:00 P.M.			
3:00 P.M.			
4:00 P.M.			
5:00 P.M.			
6:00 P.M.			
7:00 P.M.			
8:00 P.M.			
9:00 P.M.			
10:00 P.M.			
11:00 P.M.			
Midnight			

Chapter 10

My R-K-O journaling technique, first introduced in Chapter 4, offers a simple way to keep tabs on how well you're following the set point solutions. Copy the chart and put it someplace where you'll see it daily, such as in your daily planner, or on your refrigerator or bathroom mirror. But remember, the scale is your final arbiter. Don't forget to weigh yourself every morning to verify your success, whether that's losing weight or just holding steady.

R-K-O SAMPLE JOURNAL PAGE

	Mon	Tues	Wed	Thurs	Fri	Sat	Sun
Eat less							
Eat well							
Exercise							
Sleep							
Time/Life Management							
Stress Management							
Pursuit of Happiness							
OVERALL SCORE							

Eat less: Are you eating at least 450 calories at breakfast and lunch, taking twenty minutes to eat each meal, and following some of the "Nine Tips for Eating Less" (see page 94) to eat less and keep your hunger satiety score between 4 and 7?

Eat well: Are you eating plenty of fruits, vegetables, and whole grains? Do you eat fish several times per week or take a fish oil supplement? Are you steering clear of junk food?

Exercise: Are you getting thirty to sixty minutes of exercise most days of the week, including a mix of different types of activities?

Sleep: Are you getting seven to eight hours of sleep per night? Do you generally feel refreshed and energetic during the day?

Time/Life Management: Are the regular everyday chores getting done? Are you managing to find time for daily living tasks, like cleaning, maintaining your home and car, and managing your finances, as well as an hour for yourself each morning?

Stress Management: Are you taking steps to mitigate and manage stress in positive ways?

Pursuit of Happiness: Are you making enough time for yourself to relax and enjoy recreational activities? Are you trying any new classes or making time for the hobbies you already enjoy?

Selected Resources

Chapter 6

American Institute for Cancer Research (AICR)
1759 R Street NW
Washington, DC 20009
800-843-8114
www.aicr.org

You can request AIRC brochures on the following topics:

- *Moving Toward a Plant-Based Diet*

- *A Healthy Weight for Life*

- *Getting Active, Staying Active*

- *The New American Plate*

- *The New American Plate: One-Pot Meals*

- *The New American Plate: Veggies*

- *The New American Plate: Comfort Foods*

- *Homemade for Health*

- *Nutrition After Fifty*

Chapter 7

American College of Sports Medicine (ACSM)
P.O. Box 1440
Indianapolis, IN 46206-1440
317-637-9200
www.acsm.org

You can download or request brochures on how to use the following fitness aids:

- *Rubber Band Resistance Exercise*
- *Stability Balls*
- *Elliptical Trainer*
- *Free Weights*
- *Home Treadmill*
- *Personal Trainer*
- *Stair Stepper/Stair Climber*
- *Stationary Bicycles*

Arthritis Foundation
P.O. Box 7669
Atlanta, GA 30357
404-872-7100
www.arthritis.org

To find an Aquacize class in your area, click "Resources," then "Find Your Local Office."

Chapter 7

Harvard Health Publications
10 Shattuck Street
Boston, MA 02115-6011
877-649-9457
www.health.harvard.edu/special_health_reports

Harvard Health Publications puts out an excellent series of reports on health that I recommend highly. These reports, compiled by experts, include the most recent scientific evidence about a topic and offer practical recommendations. They cover a range of topics, including:

- *Exercise: A Program You Can Live With*

- *Strength and Power Training: A Guide for Adults of All Ages*

- *Improving Sleep: A Guide to a Good Night's Rest*

- *Stress Control: Techniques for Preventing and Easing Stress*

Chapter 8

National Sleep Foundation
1522 K Street NW, Suite 500
Washington, DC 20005
202-347-3471
www.sleepfoundation.org

Chapter 9

Benson-Henry Institute for Mind Body Medicine
824 Boylston Street
Chestnut Hill, MA 02467
617-732-9130
www.mbmi.org

You can order relaxation CDs via the store on their Web site, which include titles such as:

- *Healing Meditations*

- *Meditations for Personal Health and Well-Being*

- *The Tree of Awareness: Mindfulness Meditation*

- *A Collection of Relaxation Exercises*

Similar recordings are available at www.mindfulnesstapes.com/ by John Kabat-Zinn, Ph.D., a professor emeritus at the University of Massachuetts Medical School and founder of the Center for Mindfulness in Medicine, Health Care, and Society.

Chapter 10

The following resources are examples of institutions and agencies that have made positive changes to help people eat more healthfully and get more exercise.

Schools and Youth

- **The Child Nutrition and WIC Reauthorization Act of 2004** (http://www.fns.usda.gov/tn/healthy/wellnesspolicy.html) This law mandated that all schools participating in the federal school meals programs (as most do) had to develop a school wellness policy by the fall of 2006. The USDA site, above, serves as a clearinghouse of information about this policy.

- **Parents Against Junk Food** (http://www.parentsagainstjunkfood .org/) This nonprofit organization is working to ban junk food from schools.

- **Two Angry Moms** (http://www.angrymoms.org/) These two women made a documentary film that highlights some of the best (and worst) examples of school lunches. They offer other resources for getting involved in your own community.

- **The National Center for Safe Routes to School** (http://safety .fhwa.dot.gov/saferoutes/) This federal effort is helping communities make walking and bicycling to school a safe and routine activity for kids.

- **Alliance for a Healthier Generation** (http://www.healthier-generation.org/) The Alliance for a Healthier Generation, a partnership between the American Heart Association and the William J. Clinton Foundation, is a collaborative effort to stop the nationwide increase in childhood obesity by 2010. They work to transform the places that affect a child's health, including homes, schools, restaurants, doctors' offices, and the community, by forming strategic partnerships and offering tool kits for teachers, parents, kids, and companies.

Workplaces and Hospitals

- **Centers for Disease Control and Prevention, StairWELL to Better Health** (http://www.cdc.gov/nccdphp/dnpa/hwi/toolkits/ stairwell/index.htm)
  The CDC's tool kit for pleasant stairwells includes information on appearance, signage, music, tracking stair usage, and other related resources.

- **National Business Group on Health (NBGH), Promoting Healthy Weight Through Healthy Dining at Work Tool Kit** (http://www.businessgrouphealth.org/healthy/diningtoolkit.cfm)
  This tool kit helps employers assess and improve their cafeteria, vending, and catering food options. The tool kit offers information about ensuring that healthy options are available and implementing programs that provide incentives and rewards for healthy choices.

- **America's Health Insurance Plans (AHIP)** (http://www.ahip.org/)
  AHIP is a national association that represents nearly thirteen hundred member companies that provide health insurance coverage. Their goal is to help employers identify the best practices and successful strategies for minimizing health care expenses through the implementation of preventive health programs.

- **Osher Institute** (http://www.osher.hms.harvard.edu/)
  The Osher Institute is the home of the Division for Research and Education in Complementary and Integrative Medical Therapies at Harvard Medical School. One focus is helping physicians and health care providers learn about healthy foods and food preparation to better serve as healthy-eating role models and advisors.

- **Kaiser Permanente Farmers' Markets** (http://members
.kaiserpermanente.org/redirects/farmersmarkets/?rop-MRN)
Kaiser started a weekly farmers' market with organic, pesticide-
free produce from local farmers at one of its California locations
in 2003. As many as one thousand employees, physicians,
patients, and neighbors were showing up each week, leading
Kaiser to expand the markets to Kaiser locations in California,
Colorado, Georgia, and Hawaii.

Communities

- **Healthy People 2010, Healthy People in Healthy Communities
Guide** (http://www.healthypeople.gov/Publications/
HealthyCommunities2001/default.htm)
This pamphlet, released by the Department of Health and
Human Services, provides guidance for creating change in your
community. It includes tips for building community coalitions,
measuring results, and creating partnerships dedicated to
improved health.

- **Department of Health and Human Services, Healthy Women
Build Healthy Communities Tool Kit** (http://www.hrsa.gov/
WomensHealth/toolkit/menu.html)
The Department of Health and Human Services realized that
many women want to do more to improve the health of their
communities. They put together this tool kit so that women can
plan and carry out events to help others be more active and eat
more healthfully.

Notes

Chapter 1

Cardinal TM, Kaciroti N, and Lumeng JC. The figure rating scale as an index of weight status of women on videotape. *Obesity (Silver Spring)* 14 (2006): 2132–5.

Framingham Heart Study. In http://www.nhlbi.nih.gov/about/framingham/index.html (accessed May 11, 2007).

Kennedy GC. The role of depot fat in the hypothalamic control of food intake in the rat. *Proc R Soc Lond B Biol Sci* 140 (1953): 578–96.

Keys A, Brozek J, Henschel A, Mickelson O, and Taylor HL. *The Biology of Human Starvation*. Minneapolis: University of Minneapolis, 1950.

Leibel RL, Rosenbaum M, and Hirsch J. Changes in energy expenditure resulting from altered body weight. *N Engl J Med* 332 (1995): 621–8.

Salans LB, Horton ES, and Sims EA. Experimental obesity in man: cellular character of the adipose tissue. *J Clin Invest* 50 (1971): 1005–11.

Stunkard AJ, Sorensen T, and Schulsinger F. Use of the Danish Adoption Register for the study of obesity and thinness. *Res Publ Assoc Res Nerv Ment Dis* 60 (1983): 115–20.

Chapter 2

Bouchard C, Tremblay A, Despres JP, Nadeau A, Lupien PJ, Theriault G, Dussault J, Moorjani S, Pinault S, and Fournier G. The response to long-term overfeeding in identical twins. *N Engl J Med* 322 (1990): 1477–82.

Centers for Disease Control and Prevention (CDC). Trends in intake of energy and macronutrients—United States, 1971–2000. *MMWR Morb Mortal Wkly Rep* 53 (2004): 80–2.

de Castro JM, and Lilenfeld LR. Influence of heredity on dietary restraint, disinhibition, and perceived hunger in humans. *Nutrition* 21 (2005): 446–55.

Fox MK, Pac S, Devaney B, and Jankowski L. Feeding infants and toddlers study: What foods are infants and toddlers eating? *J Am Diet Assoc* 104 (2004): s22–30.

Herbert A, et al. A common genetic variant is associated with adult and child-hood obesity. *Science* 312 (2006): 279–83.

Mennella JA, Pepino MY, and Reed DR. Genetic and environmental determinants of bitter perception and sweet preferences. *Pediatrics* 115 (2005): e216–22.

Chapter 3

Beresford SA, et al. Low-fat dietary pattern and risk of colorectal cancer: the Women's Health Initiative Randomized Controlled Dietary Modification Trial. *JAMA* 295 (2006): 643–54.

Blackburn GL, and Read JL. Benefits of reducing—revisited. *Postgrad Med J* 60 (suppl 3) (1984): 13–18.

Calle EE, et al. Overweight, obesity, and mortality from cancer in a prospectively studied cohort of U.S. adults. *N Engl J Med* 348 (2003): 1625–38.

Chlebowski RT, et al. Dietary fat reduction and breast cancer outcome: interim efficacy results from the Women's Intervention Nutrition Study. *J Natl Cancer Inst* 98 (2006): 1767–76.

Diabetes Prevention Program Research Group. Reduction in the incidence of type 2 diabetes with lifestyle intervention or metformin. *N Engl J Med* 346 (2002): 393–403.

Goldstein DJ. Beneficial health effects of modest weight loss. *Int J Obes Relat Metab Disord* 16 (1992): 397–415.

Howard BV, et al. Low-fat dietary pattern and risk of cardiovascular disease: the Women's Health Initiative Randomized Controlled Dietary Modification Trial. *JAMA* 295 (2006): 655–66.

Look AHEAD Research Group. The Look AHEAD study: A description of the lifestyle intervention and the evidence supporting it. *Obesity* 14 (2006): 737–52.

Prentice AM, et al. Effects of weight cycling on body composition. *Am J Clin Nutr* 56 (1992): 209S–16S.

Prentice RL, et al. Low-fat dietary pattern and risk of invasive breast cancer: the Women's Health Initiative Randomized Controlled Dietary Modification Trial. *JAMA* 295 (2006): 629–42.

Ryan DH, et al. Look AHEAD research. Look AHEAD (Action for Health in Diabetes): design and methods for a clinical trial of weight loss for the prevention of cardiovascular disease in type 2 diabetes. *Control Clin Trials* 24 (2003): 610–28.

Weight cycling. National Task Force on the Prevention and Treatment of Obesity. *JAMA* 272 (1994): 1196–202.

Chapter 4

Eckel RH. The dietary approach to obesity; is it the diet or the disorder? *JAMA* 293 (2005): 96–7.

The Practical Guide: Identification, Evolution, and Treatment of Overweight and Obesity in Adults. NIH. Publication Number 00484, October 2000.

Wing RR, et al. A self-regulation program for maintenance of weight loss. *N Engl J Med* 355 (2006): 1563–71.

Chapter 5

Center for Science in the Public Interest. *Anyone's Guess*. Washington DC, 2003.

Dansinger ML, et al. Comparison of the Atkins, Ornish, Weight Watchers, and Zone diets for weight loss and heart disease risk reduction: a randomized trial. *JAMA* 293 (2005): 43–53.

Garner A, and Stuht J. CORE tools and patient information: easy portion-control tips for reducing calories. *Obesity Management* 1(3)(2005): 113–15.

Hudson JI, et al. The prevalence and correlates of eating disorders in the National Comorbidity Survey Replication. *Biol Psychiatry* 61 (2007): 348–58.

Ledikwe JH, et al. Dietary energy density is associated with energy intake and weight status in US adults. *Am J Clin Nutr* 83 (2006): 1362–8.

Nonas CA, and Foster GD. Setting achievable goals for weight loss. *J Am Diet Assoc* 105 (2005): S118–23.

Rolls BJ, Roe LS, and Meengs JS. Salad and satiety: energy density and portion size of a first-course salad affect energy intake at lunch. *J Am Diet Assoc* 104 (2004): 1570–6.

Rolls BJ, Roe LS, and Meengs JS. Reductions in portion size and energy density of foods are additive and lead to sustained decreases in energy intake. *Am J Clin Nutr* 83 (2006): 11–17.

Truby H, et al. Randomised controlled trial of four commercial weight loss programmes in the UK: initial findings from the BBC "diet trials." *BMJ* 332 (2006): 1309–14.

Wansink B, and Chandon P. Meal size, not body size, explains errors in estimating the calorie content of meals. *Ann Intern Med* 145 (2006): 326–32.

Wansink B, van Ittersum K, and Painter JE. Ice cream illusions bowls, spoons, and self-served portion sizes. *Am J Prev Med* 31 (2006): 240–3.

Westenhoefer J, Stunkard AJ, and Pudel V. Validation of the flexible and rigid control dimensions of dietary restraint. *Int J Eat Disord* 26 (1999): 53–64.

Williamson DA, et al. Effects of consuming mycoprotein, tofu or chicken upon subsequent eating behaviour, hunger and safety. *Appetite* 46 (2006): 41–8.

Chapter 6
Appel LJ, et al. A clinical trial of the effects of dietary patterns on blood pressure. DASH Collaborative Research Group. *N Engl J Med* 336 (1997): 1117–24.

Block G. Foods contributing to energy intake in the US: data from NHANES III and NHANES 1999–2000. *Journal of Food Composition and Analysis* 17, no. 3–4 (2004): 439–47.

Kris-Etherton PM, et al. Fish consumption, fish oil, omega-3 fatty acids and cardiovascular disease. *Circulation* 106 (2002): 2747–57.

Subar AF, et al. Dietary sources of nutrients among US adults, 1989 to 1991. *J Am Diet Assoc* 98 (1998): 537–47.

United States Department of Agriculture. *Let's Eat Out: Americans weigh taste, convenience, and nutrition* (2006).

Chapter 7
Elder SJ, and Roberts SB. The effects of exercise on food intake and body fatness: a summary of published studies. *Nutr Rev* 65 (2007): 1–19.

Levine JA, and Miller J. The energy expenditure of using a "walk-and-work" desk for office-workers with obesity. *Br J Sports Med* 41 (2007): 558–61.

Chapter 8
Jacobs GD, et al., Cognitive behavior therapy and pharmacotherapy for insomnia: a randomized controlled trial and direct comparison. *Arch Intern Med* 164 (2004): 1888–96.

Saper CB, Scammell TE, and Lu J. Hypothalamic regulation of sleep and circadian rhythms. *Nature* 437 (2005): 1257–63.

Chapter 9
Benson H. *The Relaxation Response*. New York: HarperCollins Publishers, Inc., 2000.

Brownell KD. *The LEARN Program for Weight Control*. Dallas, Texas: American Health Publishing Company, 1991.

Dallman MF, Pecoraro NC, and la Fleur SE. Chronic stress and comfort foods: self-medication and abdominal obesity. *Brain Behav Immun* 19 (2005): 275–80.

Dallman MF, et al. Chronic stress and obesity: a new view of "comfort food." *Proc Natl Acad Sci USA* 100 (2003): 11696–701.

Hallowell EM. *Connect: 12 Vital Ties That Open Your Heart, Lengthen Your Life, and Deepen Your Soul.* Pocket, 2001.

Garg N, et al. The influence of incidental affects in consumers' food intake. *Journal of Marketing* 71 (2007): 194–206.

Seligman M. Positive psychology: an introduction. *American Psychologist* 55 (2000): 5–14.

Shaw K, et al. Psychological interventions for overweight or obesity. *Cochrane Database of Systematic Reviews* 18 (2005): CD003818

Wadden TA, and Foster GD. Weight and Lifestyle Inventory (WALI). *Surg Obes Relat Dis* 2 (2006): 180–99.

Chapter 10

Canales M, et al. Supermarket price check—healthy can be less expensive! *Today's Dietician* 8 (2006): 50.

Wing RR, and Phelan S. Long-term weight loss maintenance. *Am J Clin Nutr* 82 (suppl 1) (2005): 222S–5S.

Index

mindfulness, 86, 185
Minnesota Starvation Study, 10–12
Monell Chemical Senses Center, 19
morning meals, 82–83, 99, 192, 208–11
motivation, 136
motivational interviewing (MI), 72
mouth hunger, 178
movie stars, 14
movie theater popcorn, 31
multivitamins, *107*, 123–24
muscles, 64, 143, 148
music, 138

National Center of Complementary and
    Alternative Medicine, 158
National Health and Nutrition Examina-
    tion Survey, 32–33
National Heart, Lung, and Blood
    Institute, *94*
National Institutes of Health (NIH), 74,
    75
National Sleep Foundation (NSF),
    152–53, 155
National Weight Control Registry
    (NWCR), 58, 191–93
natural selection, 22
NEAT (nonexercise activity thermogen-
    esis), 132, 137
nervous system, 130
New American Plate, 103
nicotine, 24, 155
nonbenzodiazepine hypnotics, 159
nonexercise activity thermogenesis
    (NEAT), 132, 137
norepinephrine (noradrenaline), 197
nortriptyline (Aventyl, Pamelor), 159
nurses, 73
nutrition labels, 83, 118–20, *119*
nuts, 106, *107*, 113

oatmeal, 113
obesity
    and blood pressure, 47–48
    and cancer, 50
    defined, 18, 23
    and heart disease, 10
    as metabolic disease, 9
offices, 133

oils, 106, 110, 116
olive oil, 110
omega-3 fatty acids, 124, *125*
Optifast, 196
orlistat (Xenical), 196–97
Ornish diet, 81
osteoporosis, 143
ovarian cancer, 50
overeating, 31
overstimulation, 155
overweight, defined, 18, 23

palm-sized portions, 93
Pamelor (nortriptyline), 159
pancreas, 7
pancreatic cancer, 50
pantry staples, *207–8*
parenthood, 26, 155
Parkinson's disease, 130
parties, 96, 97, 121
pasta, 92, 112
patient-oriented treatment, 71–72
peanuts, 106
pear-shape body types, 46
peas, 106
pedometers, 60, 62, 136, 138–39, 147
pepperoni pizza, *94*
perceived hunger, 20, 86
perspiration, 8
phentermine (Adipex-P), 197
physical activity
    active lifestyle described, 128–29
    and body mass index (BMI), 75
    compared to exercise, 131–33 (*see also*
        exercise)
    developing a routine, 136–43
    and heart disease, 10
    importance of, 43, 191–92
    increasing, *134*
    and metabolism, 5, 131
    opportunities for, 15
    and pedometers, 60, 62, 136, 138–39,
        147 (*see also* walking)
    recommendations for, 127
    recording activity levels, 59–61
    in schools, 26
    types of, 131–32
physical therapists, 73, 148

picnic plates, 103
plant-based fats, 106, *107*
plant-based proteins, 112
plateau periods, 44, *45*
plates, *85*, 95, 103–5, *104, 105*
popcorn, 31, 112
pork, 112
portions
    and dining out, 30, 31, 121
    gauging portion sizes, 92–93
    oversized portions, 15, 83, *94*
    and plates, 95, 103–5, *104, 105*
    portion distortion, 30, 76, 91–94, 99
positive psychology, 183
Post, 99
potassium *108*, 108
potatoes, *108*
pot-luck dinners, 98
poultry, *107*, 112, 116
Powerade, 142
pre-eating, 97
pregnancy, 2, 4, 24, 26, 34
premature death, 51
Prentice, Andrew, 17
primary care providers (PCP), 70–73
processed foods, 102, *102*
progressive muscle relaxation, 179
Prosom (estazolam), 159
prostate cancer, 50, 124
protein diets, 79, 81
proteins, 106, 112–13, 120
prune juice, *108*
psychologists, 73
psychotherapy, 181

Quaker Weight Control Oatmeal, 113
quinoa, 112

ramelteon (Rozerem), 159
rate of weight loss, 41
rebounds in weight, 40, 47
recipes, evaluation of, 116
rectal cancer, 50
red meat, *107*
reduced-fat foods, *32*
refined starches, 106, *107*, 107, 110
resistance training, 133, 141–43. *See also* exercise

restaurants. *See* dining out
resting energy expenditure (REE), 4, 19
Restoril (temazepam), 159
rice, 112
rigid control of eating, 88–89, 193
rimonabant, 197
ritual eating, 16
R-K-O journaling, 59–61, 79, 114, 195, 235
roasting, 116
Rockefeller University, 13–14
Roux-en-Y gastric by-pass procedure, xiii
Rozerem (ramelteon), 159
running, 141, 142, 148

salads, 97, 109, 110
salt, 107–8, 110
sandwiches, 110
satiety, 6, 21, 98, 120
saturated fats, 118
sautéing, 116
scales, 58–59, 192
schools, 25–26
sedentary lifestyle, 127–28, 137–38
Seligman, Martin E. P., 169, 183, 184
sensory-specific satiety, 98
set point
    changes in, 1–2, 3–4
    defined, 1
    maintenance of weight, 43–44
    summary of weight-loss cycle, 63–66
    See also 10% rule
sex, 4, 130
shellfish, *125*
shoes for walking, 62
shopping for groceries, 97, 114, 118, 207–8
sibutramine (Meridia), 196
silhouettes
    charts, *3*
    described, 2
    identifying your silhouette, 65–70, *67–70*
    and preparations for program, 63
    and weight changes, 3, 18
single-food diets, 98
single-serving snack bags, 114
sit-down meals, 120

skipping meals, 121
sleep
    average requirements for, 152
    distractions from, 160–62
    and exercise, 130, 155–56
    guidelines for, 156
    habits, 54–55, 57
    importance of, 43, 44, 152–53
    napping, 153
    sleep apnea, 75, 157–58, 198
    and stress, 154, 155, 157, 176
    and time management, 151–52,
        160–61, *161*, 163–65, *164–65*
    treating sleep issues, 157–60
    and weight, 36, 46, 153–55
SlimFast shakes, xiii, 98
smoking, 10, 24, 28, 50, 75
smoothies, 109
snacks
    and children, *25*
    costs of, 194
    and dining out, *30*
    options for, 117
    and portion control, 93
    and "pre-eating," 97
    prior to going out, 121
    and sleep, 155
    strategies for, 78
Snickers test, 21
social workers, 73
sodium, 107–8, 118
Sonata (zaleplon), 159
soups, 97
soy products, 113
speed of weight loss, 12
spinach, *108*
sprints, 141
stability balls, 133
stair climbing, 141, 166
Stanford Institute for the Quantitative
    Study of Society, 161–62
starvation, xiii, 11–12, 22, 40, 47
statistics on successful weight loss, 40
stimulants, 155, 156
stomach, 7–8
stomach cancer, 50
*Strength and Power Training: A Guide for
    Adults of all Ages*, 143

strength training, 133, 139, 142–43,
    192. *See also* exercise
stress, 169–85
    dealing with, 176–83
    and disinhibition, 86
    and emotional eating, 36, 172,
        176–77, *177*
    external and internal stressors,
        174
    inventory of, 55
    perceived stress, *175–76*
    and physical activity, 130, 136, 138,
        145
    responses to, 173
    and sleep, 154, 155, 157, 176
    traumatic stressors, 173
    and weight maintenance, 43
stretching, 138
strokes, 27, 48, 49, 103, 130
substitutions, *102*, 116
suburban neighborhoods, 35
sugar, 32, *32*, 110, 119
suicide, 172
Super Size Me, 30
supplements for weight loss, 5, 39–40,
    123
surgeries, weight-loss, xiii, 7, 75, *75*,
    198–99
sweets, 80, 89–90

Tai chi, 145
teeth, brushing, 78, 90
television cooking shows, 115
television viewing, 32–33, 161, 162–63,
    176
temazepam (Restoril), 159
temperature, body, 6
10% rule, 37–51
    benefits of, 45–51
    calorie chart, *42*
    described, 41–43
    maintenance of weight, 66
    repeating the cycle, 43, 66
    studies on, 13–14
thighs, 46
thirst, 22, 34, 90
thumb-tip portion sizes, 93
thyroid conditions, 5, 27